A COMPLETE GUIDE TO
UNDERSTANDING AND PRACTISING

YOGA

SUE LILLY

Published in 2001 by Caxton Editions
20 Bloomsbury Street
London WC1B 3JH
a member of the Caxton Publishing Group

© copyright 2001 Caxton Publishing Group
Reprint 2002 , 2003
Designed and produced for Caxton Editions
by Open Door Limited

Editing: Mary Morton
Typesetting: Julie Payne
Illustration: Andrew Shepherd, Art Angle
Digital Imagery © copyright 2001 Photodisc, Inc.

Title: YOGA
ISBN: 1-84067-289-7

IMPORTANT NOTICE

This book is not intended to be a substitute for medical advice or
treatment. Any person with a condition requiring medical
attention should consult a qualified medical practitioner or
suitable therapist.

A COMPLETE GUIDE TO
UNDERSTANDING AND PRACTISING

YOGA

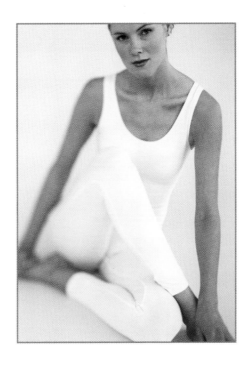

SUE LILLY

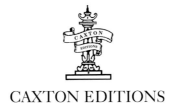

CAXTON EDITIONS

CONTENTS

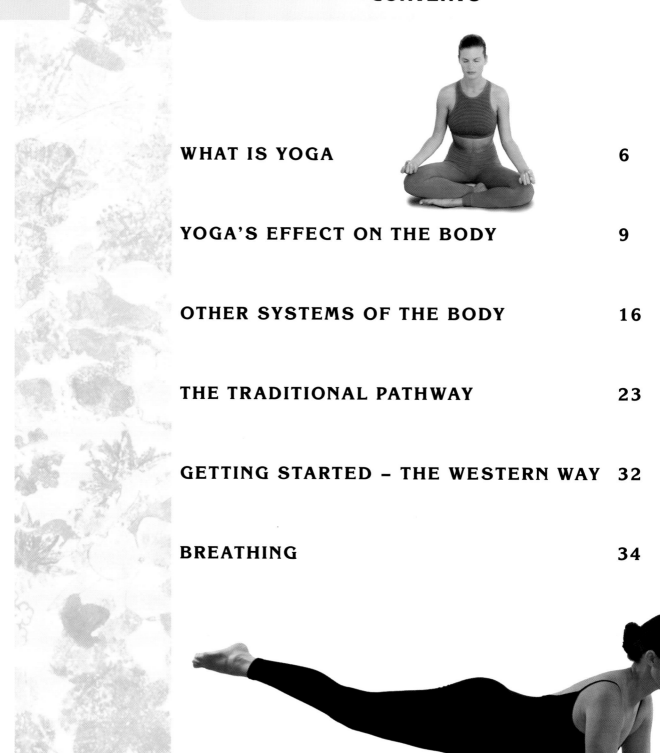

CONTENTS

WHAT IS YOGA?

"Yoga" comes from the root word "yuj" in Sanskrit, meaning "to join with" or "to harness".

Yoga is a practice. It is not a religion and not necessarily a philosophy, though there are many books around on just those aspects.

It has its roots in India, thousands of years ago, and is probably the oldest system of holistic health in the world. It is as valid today, as it ever was, maybe more so, as we juggle the pressures of life in the 21st century with our physical, emotional, mental and spiritual needs.

Right: Shiva the Hindu god, said to be the founder of Yoga.

Far right: Yoga is as valid today, as it ever was, maybe more so, as we juggle the pressures of life in the 21st century with our physical, emotional, mental and spiritual needs.

The ancient practitioners of yoga, yogis, developed a deep understanding of what we humans are really all about. They observed the interaction we have with one another and with the environment, and devised many ways to explain what they saw. The physical body was seen to be the vehicle of the human being. Using the modern analogy of a car, the mind is then the driver. The complex combination that gives the car its ability to travel is seen as the soul, or the core of the person. All aspects of the vehicle need to be working harmoniously for forward motion to occur. In this way, the yogis placed the mind in context with the rest of the being, notably NOT as the core of the person. Their observations also led to the realisation that physical movement and breathing techniques helped to steady the function of the mind. Ancient Sanskrit texts were first translated in the early nineteenth century. Unfortunately, as often happens, the bias of those doing the translation, affected the translation. At that time it was perceived that the philosophy and practice revealed in these texts belonged to a culture that was far less evolved than that in the Western world, and therefore had nothing to offer.

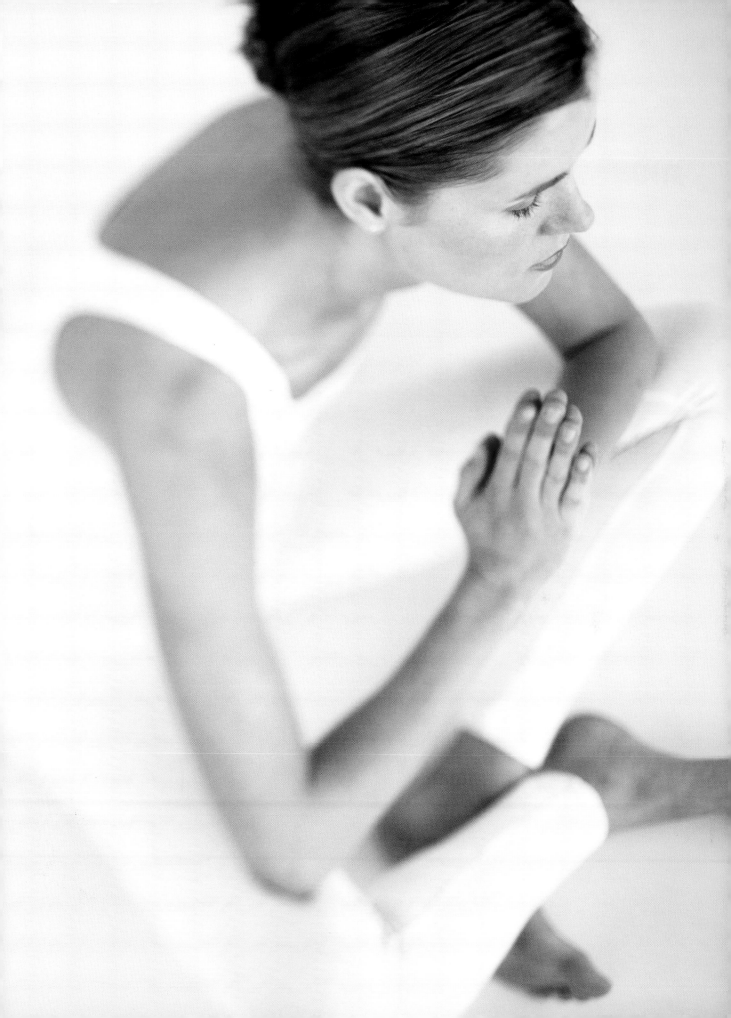

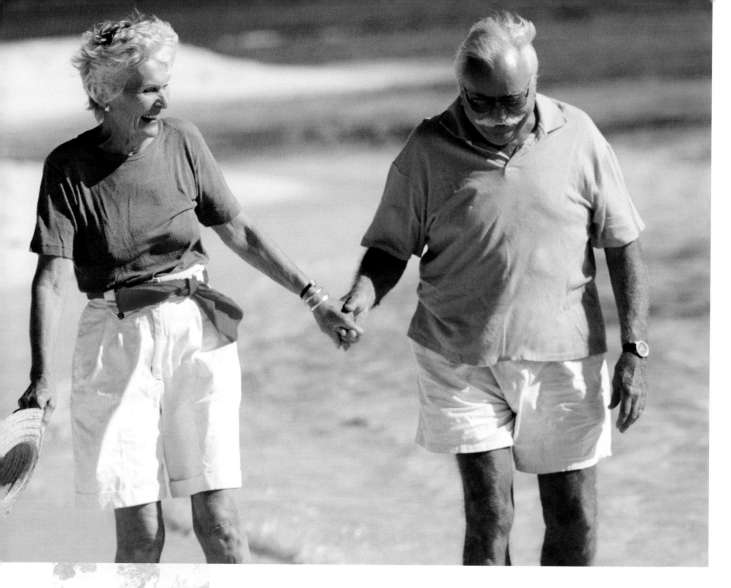

Above: many psychologists and psychiatrists recognise that if more of us practised yoga we would be healthier happier and live longer, and these are just a few of the benefits to be gained.

Science and physical discovery were in full flood, and the subtleties of yogic practices were not appreciated or seen to have any validity.

Many philosophers, psychologists and psychiatrists today, however, recognise that if more of us practised yoga we would be:

- *healthier*
- *happier*
- *live longer*
- *content with fewer of the things we don't really need*

Our society would also be more caring and respectful and it is likely that there would be less violence in the world.

Fortunately, nowadays we have access to translations that are truer approximations to the original texts and there have now been several generations of yoga practitioners in the West. It is hoped that this book will act as a straightforward guide to those wishing to introduce yoga into their lives.

For yoga to do its job of uniting the many different parts of ourselves and harnessing our energy to create a whole person, its effect needs to reach every aspect of our being.

This is why the observances of the traditional practice of yoga include the communal and personal ethics of everyday living. (For detailed explanation see 'The Traditional Pathway' p. 23)

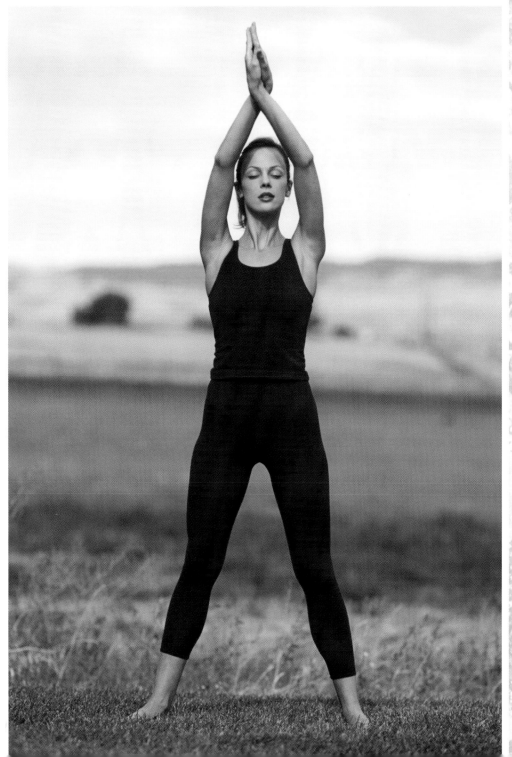

Left: the aim of yoga is to harness the many different parts of ourselves to create a whole person.

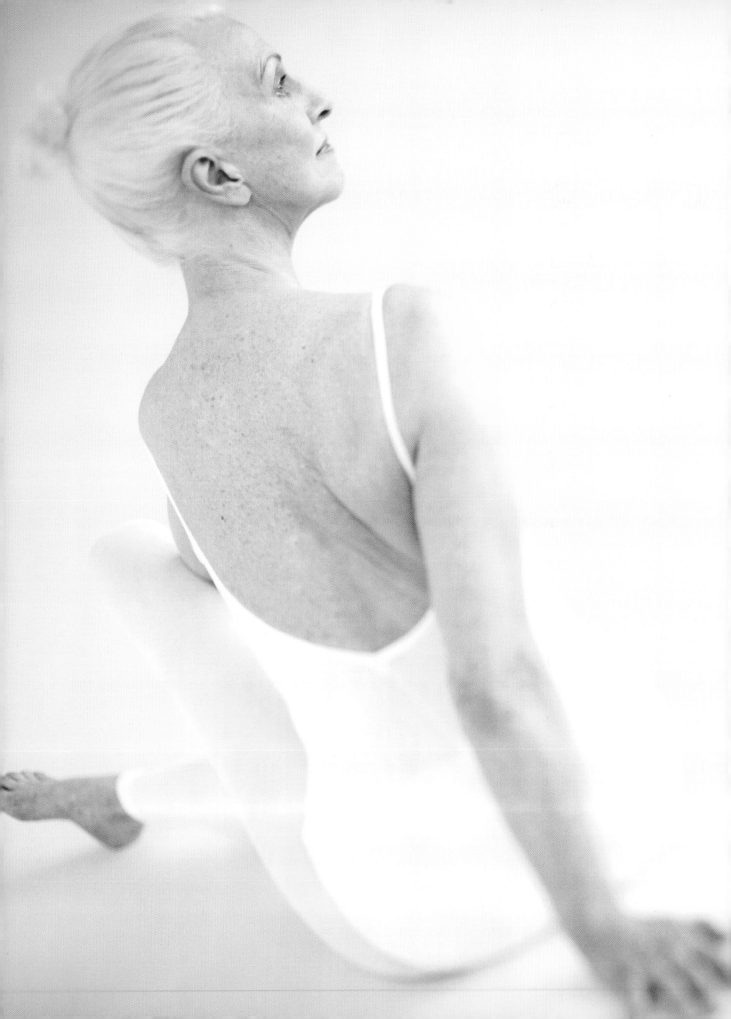

PHYSICAL

The life-giving quality of food was recognised by the ancients as a cornerstone to wholeness – an idea that is again being taken up by more and more people today.

Diet provides our bodies with the necessary nutrition and fuel to maintain health and activity. What we eat is often governed by the society in which we live, and by the local climate and conditions where we live. We also acquire personal habits and preferences. The more aware we become of the need to provide ourselves with good nutrition, the more we may find that we step away from the restraints and traditions of our upbringing. Yoga philosophy points out that it is necessary to be aware that different foods vary in the life-force that they provide. This can include food grown without pesticides and artificial fertilisers, but it also covers the types of food we eat.

People beginning yoga practices can sometimes find the regimes suggested in books or by teachers to be harsh, difficult or unacceptable. If these regimes are given as a pre-requisite to starting yoga practice, they can be very disheartening or off-putting. Given the choice, people who have practised yoga for a while will often make changes of their own accord.

The physical exercise provided by the postures or asanas helps the mechanics of the body in several ways.

Gently moving through the different postures will stretch and relax the ligaments and muscles. When performing postures, good practice is to move or stretch until some discomfort begins, hold that position for a few breaths, and then return to the first position.

This keeps your actions in tune with the sensing mechanism of the muscles (the Schwann cells around the nerve fibres and the Golgi mechanisms in cells). If you habitually push the muscles and ligaments over the boundaries created by these sensing mechanisms, it may result in better looking postures and gymnastic excellence, but it completely loses sight of what yoga is really about.

Left: the gentle action of yoga can be practised safely and provide many benefits to pregnant women (above) and elderly people (far left).

Breathing exercises can be, for many people, the single most important health-giving practice that yoga encourages. Few of us really breathe properly. Without good breathing habits we starve our body of life-giving oxygen (the inbreath), whilst depriving our body of an efficient way to remove waste products (the outbreath).

Considering how vital breathing is, it is surprising that more is not done to teach people to make better use of it. After all, if you stop to think about it, we can go without food for weeks, without water for days – but we can only survive without air for a few minutes.

Breathing has three main physical functions: it allows the body to distribute oxygen to all the organs and the brain;

it automatically creates a means to expel waste carbon dioxide from the body; it enables us to direct and control the flow of energy around the body.

Relaxation is crucial to the maintenance of good health. As the body relaxes, the most important physical benefit is the increase of blood flow to every part of the system, bringing oxygen and nutrients to the cells and speeding up the removal of their waste products.

At first sight, meditation may not appear to have any physical effects. However, meditation augments relaxation and creates peace both in the mind and the emotions which enables the body to "be" rather than "do". We live in a society that gauges an individual's value by what we "do". This view creates a lot of pressure to perform, succeed and usually over-work. It is very easy to lose touch with ourselves and just to be still. Taking time out to experience "just being" gives the opportunity for very deep healing to occur on all levels.

Far right: relaxation is crucial to the maintenance of good health. Taking time out of a hectic modern lifestyle allows the opportunity for deep healing to occur on all levels.

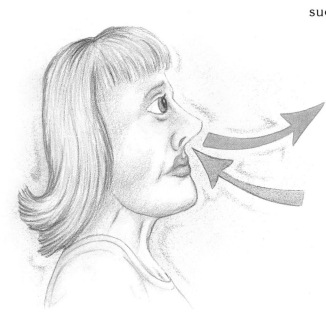

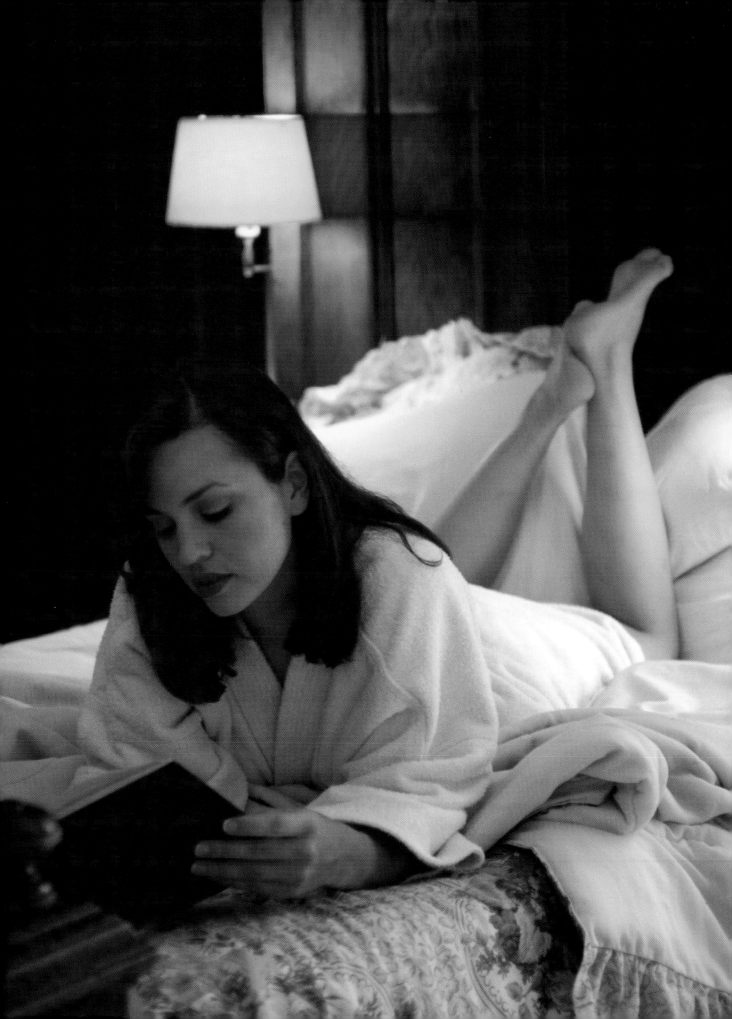

EMOTIONAL AND MENTAL

The emotional and mental effects of yoga practice are consistent from all viewpoints, for each aspect of the practice calms very effectively. For example, if the observances are followed concerning food, blood sugar levels become more stable, which in turn reduces any tendency to have mood swings and depression.

Thinking patterns and thought processes are also affected by all aspects of yoga practice. Personal attitudes and behaviour patterns can be examined and given a useful framework by the ethics and observances.

The postures help to focus the mental awareness of the physical body and allow the physical systems to slow down.

The breathing exercises bring peace to the mind and quickly reduce mental overload.

Relaxation techniques also help to quieten the mind and reduce our tendency to become distracted by the slightest outside noise or activity.

Meditation techniques introduce perspective and clarity to every level of life, but particularly to the thinking processes. Meditation creates the opportunity to place everyday life in a more universal or spiritual context.

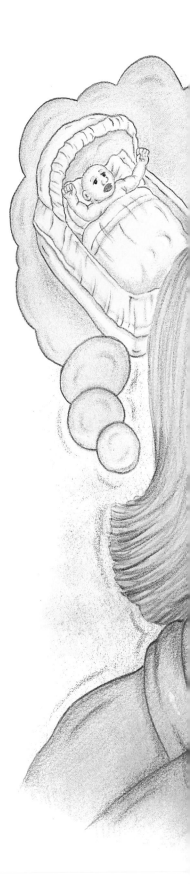

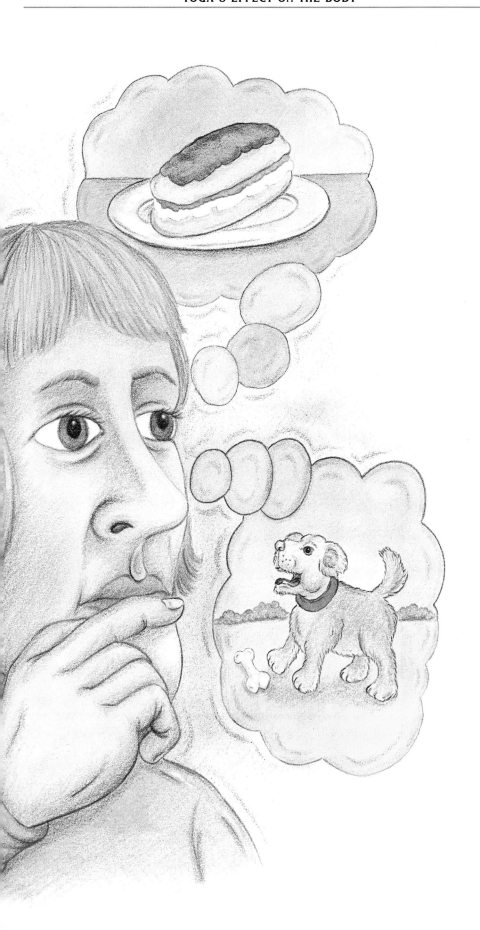

OTHER SYSTEMS OF THE BODY

CHAKRAS AND NADIS

Yoga also works with the systems of the body that we in the West are less familiar with. These energy models were introduced to Westerners in the early part of the twentieth century by writers like C.W. Leadbetter, although diagrams have been found in works dating back to the late seventeenth century.

Sushuma

Ida

Pingala

Ancient tradition holds that there are numerous invisible channels around and inside the body of a living person. Through these channels, or "nadis", flows the life-force, known in India as "prana" and in China as "chi". It is said that there are around 72,000 nadis, though three nadis are regarded as the most important conduits for prana.

First there is the Sushumna, or central channel, which follows the line of the spinal cord, up the backbone. Two others, the Ida and Pingala which also start at the base of the spine, ascend on either side of the Sushumna and cross over in several places along the length of the spine.

Where nadis cross each other, an energy vortex is formed. These vortices are known as chakras or wheels.

There are thousands of chakras throughout the subtle energy system. However, those created by the crossing of Ida and Pingala on the Sushumna are the most significant. There are six located on the Sushumna, with a seventh located just above the head.

Each of the chakras can be described by their functions and correspondences and they have direct links to the endocrine glands in the body.

It must be remembered, though, that the chakras are part of a complex interdependent system, and do not function in isolation.

Looking through the functions and correspondences, you may realise that there are one or more chakras, where you feel your energy does not function particularly well. It is quite usual for there to be strengths and weaknesses in each individual's makeup. When you begin to practise the postures or asanas, you may find that the ones relating to those chakras are more difficult for you.

Although you may focus on a particular posture to help that chakra, it is important to realise that this needs to be seen in context with the system as a whole. All postures in the sequence should be attempted.

Similarly, with chakras that are working well there is often a correlation that the corresponding postures are easy to do. Be careful not to fall into the trap of concentrating only on those postures that are easy and enjoyable for you.

The postures each have a focus on one or more chakra. The sequences in this book work systematically with the whole of the system and are therefore balancing to each chakra and to the body as a whole.

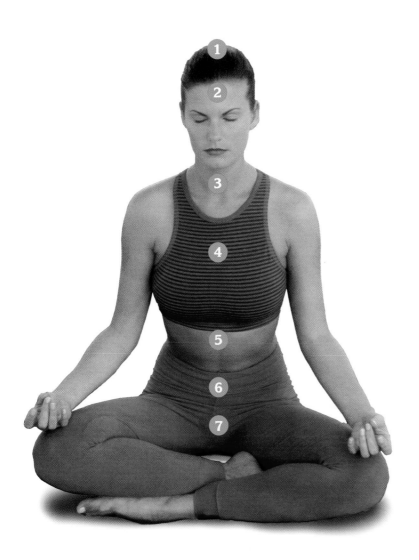

1 crown chakra – sahasrara
2 brow chakra – ajna
3 throat chakra – visuddha
4 heart chakra – anahata,
5 solar plexus chakra – manipura,
6 sacral chakra – svadistana,
7 base chakra – muladhara

FUNCTIONS AND CORRESPONDENCES OF THE CHAKRAS

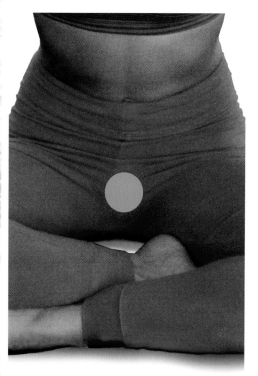

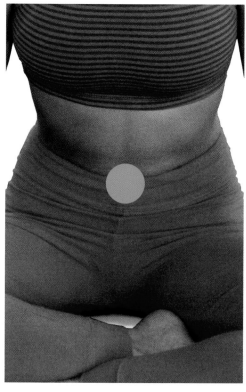

**BASE CHAKRA –
MULADHARA, MEANING "ROOT"**

**SACRAL CHAKRA – SVADISTANA,
MEANING "SWEETNESS"**

Position: base of the spine
Element: earth
Glands: adrenals
Physical: survival energy,
blood, activity, motivation,
movement
Emotional: anger, passion,
assertiveness, enthusiasm,
feeling secure
Mental: ability to initiate
projects, business skills
Spiritual: protection and links
with the planet and reality

Position: behind and below the
navel
Element: water
Gland: reproductive
Physical: sense of touch,
excretion, large intestine,
bladder, kidneys
Emotional: ability to let go,
pleasure, desire
Mental: artistry, practical ideas,
creativity
Spiritual: flow of energy
through nadis, being protective

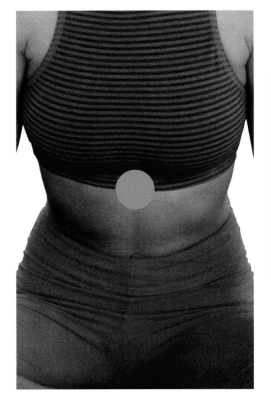

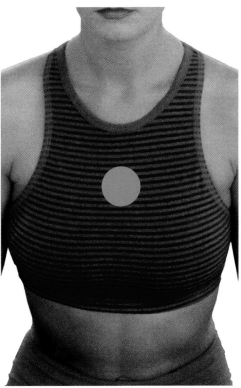

SOLAR PLEXUS CHAKRA — MANIPURA, MEANING "LUSTROUS GEM"

HEART CHAKRA — ANAHATA, MEANING "UNSTRUCK"

Position: below the ribcage
Element: fire
Glands: pancreas
Physical: digestion, immune system, liver, gallbadder, pancreas, small intestine stomach, skin, (also kidneys)
Emotional: happiness, joy, contentment, fear, anxiety, terror
Mental: logic, clarity, discrimination, worry
Spiritual: knowledge of true self, feeling of belonging

Position: centre of the sternum (breastbone)
Element: air
Gland: thymus
Physical: lungs, heart, arms, hands, breathing
Emotional: caring, loving, sharing, relating, keeping perspective and boundaries, envy
Mental: independence, space, freedom, balance, ability to organise
Spiritual: following your own path, doing your own thing

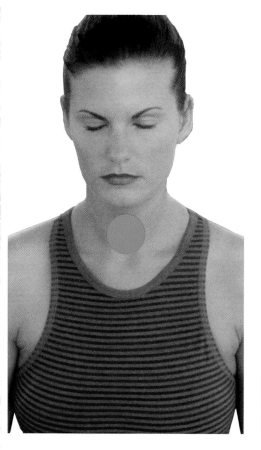

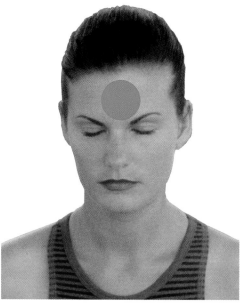

THROAT CHAKRA – VISUDDHA, MEANING "PURITY"

BROW CHAKRA – AJNA, MEANING "TO PERCEIVE"

Position: throat
Element: ether
Gland: thyroid, parathyroid
Physical: neck, throat, thyroid, ear, nose, communication, flow of energy
Emotional: calm, detachment, loyalty, peacefulness
Mental: teaching, philosophy, idealism
Spiritual: channelling, clear communication

Position: centre of forehead, above and between the eyes
Element: light
Gland: pineal
Physical: forehead, eyes
Emotional: isolation, security in self
Mental: intuition, perception
Spiritual: synthesis, seeing patterns

KUNDALINI

A little above the base of the spine is a store of dormant energy, called kundalini. This energy remains dormant in most people. Yoga, meditation and spiritual practices will eventually activate this energy. When this happens, it infuses the individual with drive and insight as regards their spiritual goals.

Some people begin yoga under the misapprehension that they must activate their kundalini and concentrate on that as the only goal. There are, however, plenty of casualties throughout history that suggest that this is inadvisable. The body's physical, emotional, mental and spiritual states need to be clear and developed enough to be able to handle the powerful creativity released. Premature activation can be like blowing an irreplaceable major fuse in an electrical circuit – the whole system fails. Since kundalini activates naturally as part of human development it is wise to see its activation as a pointer to progress along the way, not as the target.

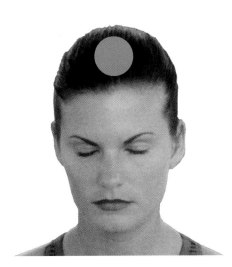

CROWN CHAKRA – SAHASRARA, MEANING "THOUSAND-PETALLED"

Position: *above the top of the head*
Element: *thought*
Gland: *pituitary*
Physical: *brain, nervous systems, spinal cord, co-ordination*
Emotional: *bliss, confusion, escapism*
Mental: *meditation, learning difficulties*
Spiritual: *links with the Infinite*

Below: Since kundalini, located at the base of the spine, activates naturally as part of human development it is wise to see its activation as a pointer to progress along the way, not as the target.

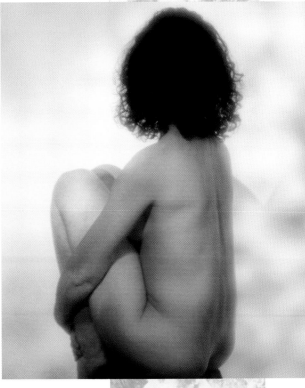

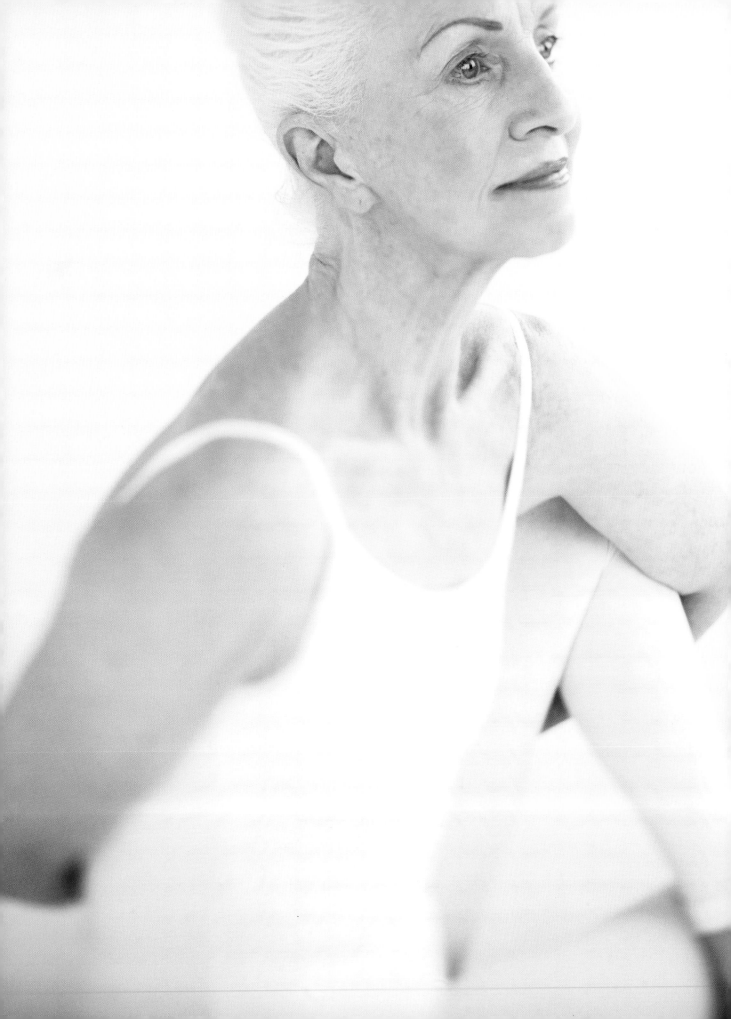

Yoga, in its most traditional format, is called "the eight-fold path", which is also sometimes referred to as Raja or Astanga yoga.

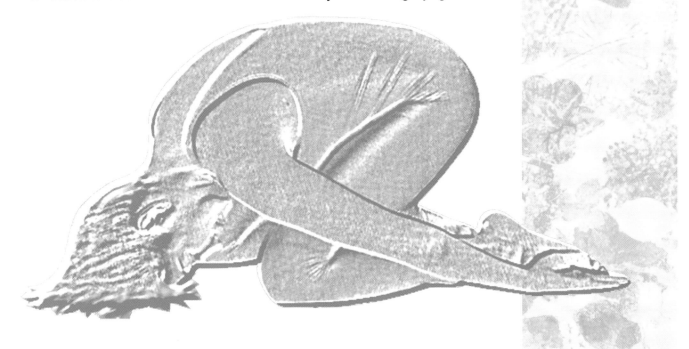

THE EIGHT LIMBS OF YOGA

The names of each of the steps (sometimes known as "limbs") are as follows:

The first three are grouped together as outward quests, challenges or tasks:

Yama
– *general behaviour*

Niyama
– *personal ethics and conduct*

Asana
– *postures.*

The next two are inner practices:

Pranayama
– *breathing techniques;*

Pratyahara
– *sense withdrawal or sense control.*

The final three are seen as quests for the soul:

Dharana
– *concentration*

Dhyana
– *meditation*

Samadhi
– *union.*

Students studying yoga in a traditional setting would start with yama and niyama. After several years cultivating the appropriate way of thinking and behaving, students would then begin to practise asanas or postures. After some time with postures, the students would begin to include pranayama, and each succeeding element.

The goal of each of these steps is to prepare a person for meditation and to clear the subtle pathways of the body to allow energy to flow more easily, so that meditation leads to samadhi.

Yama is subdivided into five disciplines that are said to be the foundation of an ethical society and are therefore very general in their guidance.

1. Ahimsa

This is often translated as non-violence. It is, however, a very broad concept, not restricted simply to avoiding killing or destroying.

Traditional texts emphasise that ahimsa is primarily a state of mind which applies to any area of life. It is stated that fear and anger are the causes that drive people to be violent.

To survive, everything must eat something else – be it vegetables, fruit or meat.

Our personal attitude to how and what we do is the crucial aspect of ahimsa. Criticising ourselves or others for what we may judge to be shortcomings of ahimsa is as much violence as any physical destruction.

2. Satya

Satya is translated as "truth". This is not limited only to telling or speaking the truth. Satya also advises against swearing, telling tales, gossiping and ridiculing people's values and beliefs.

Right: Ahimsa, often translated as nonviolence is a broad concept which relates to the mental and spiritual violence as well as the more obvious physical violence which occurs in modern-day society.

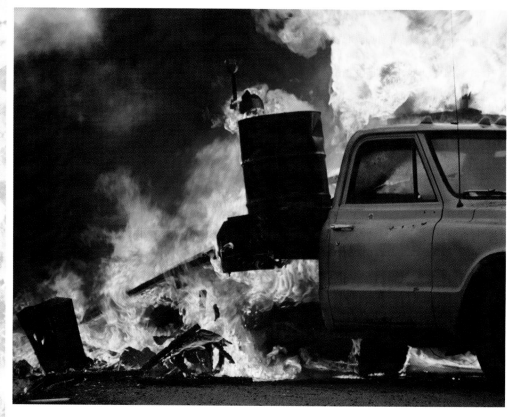

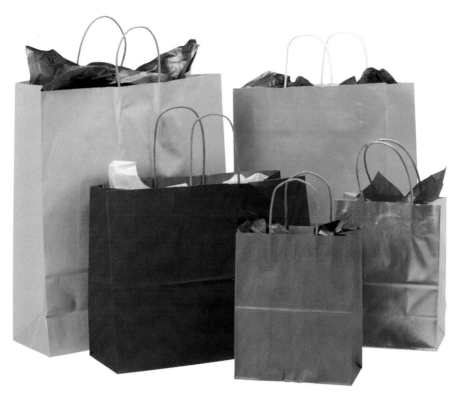

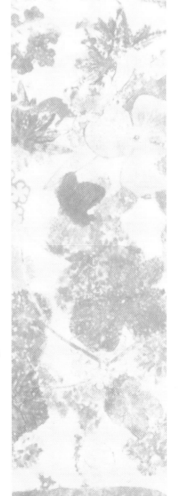

Left: asteya includes the desire to acquire material things, that is, craving for things we do not really need.

3. Asteya

Asteya can be described as covetousness and all the degrees between vague envy and actually stealing what belongs to someone else. Like all other yamas, this operates on many levels. It covers misuse of anything, anyone and loss of trust. The concept of asteya also includes the desire to acquire material things, that is, craving for things we do not really need.

4. Brahmacharya

This describes self-restraint and celibacy. Commentaries on the ancient texts present different views from the broad "seeing the divine in all creation" to emphasising the need for continence in all aspects of life. The fundamental quality of brahmacharya is respect and good management of resources.

5. Aparigraha

This relates to the tendency to hoard and collect what is not immediately required. It is related, in part, to asteya (non-stealing). It centres around whether we have faith that we have all we need to live. The phrase "Live simply – that all may simply live" sums up aparigraha. The more complex our lives, the more we fear loss or change. The more we fear loss or change, the less we are inclined to grow spiritually.

NIYAMA
These five observances are more applicable to individual and personal behaviour.

1. Saucha
This is translated as purity of the body. All aspects of the eight-fold path of yoga lead to purifying the various aspects of the body. This niyama is often thought to focus primarily on food.

Food in the West has become quite a complicated issue. The traditional Indian approach would be to aim to eat a simple, organic, vegetarian diet. The basic idea is that the purer your food, the purer your body becomes. "Rubbish in – rubbish out" and "You are what you eat" are both maxims that describe saucha. The oldest of texts, however, point out that all the yamas are applicable to this section and they also recognise that a sudden change in eating habits can be very harmful. Saucha also covers the purity and cleanliness of where you eat and also of where you do your spiritual practice and meditation.

2. Santosha
Contentment or santosha is a balanced outlook on life and begins to appear after a lot of work to understand ourselves. The mind cannot be a means to union without contentment. Tranquillity, peace, happiness and joy need to be cultivated for well-being.

3. Tapas
The words purification, self-discipline and austerity can create unease in many Westerners. In traditional yoga they are regarded as qualities to build character. Tapas is the unstinting effort to apply the yamas in all aspects of life.

4. Svadhyaya
This covers study and learning, but it is at its most relevant when dealing with self-reflection and self-awareness. On one level, we can study the sacred texts. To embrace the niyama fully, though, we can keep a personal, reflective journal or diary, highlighting our philosophical views on life as they change during the practice of yoga and the study of the philosophy behind yoga.

5. Isvara pranidhana
This is the dedication of all activity and fruits of activity to higher divine forces, whatever suits our own spiritual or religious beliefs. This helps us remain detached from the results of our actions, and from becoming proud as a result of the praise we may receive from others. Isvara pranidhana maintains a balanced perspective on life.

Right: Saucha is often thought to focus primarily on food. The basic idea is that the purer your food, the purer your body becomes.

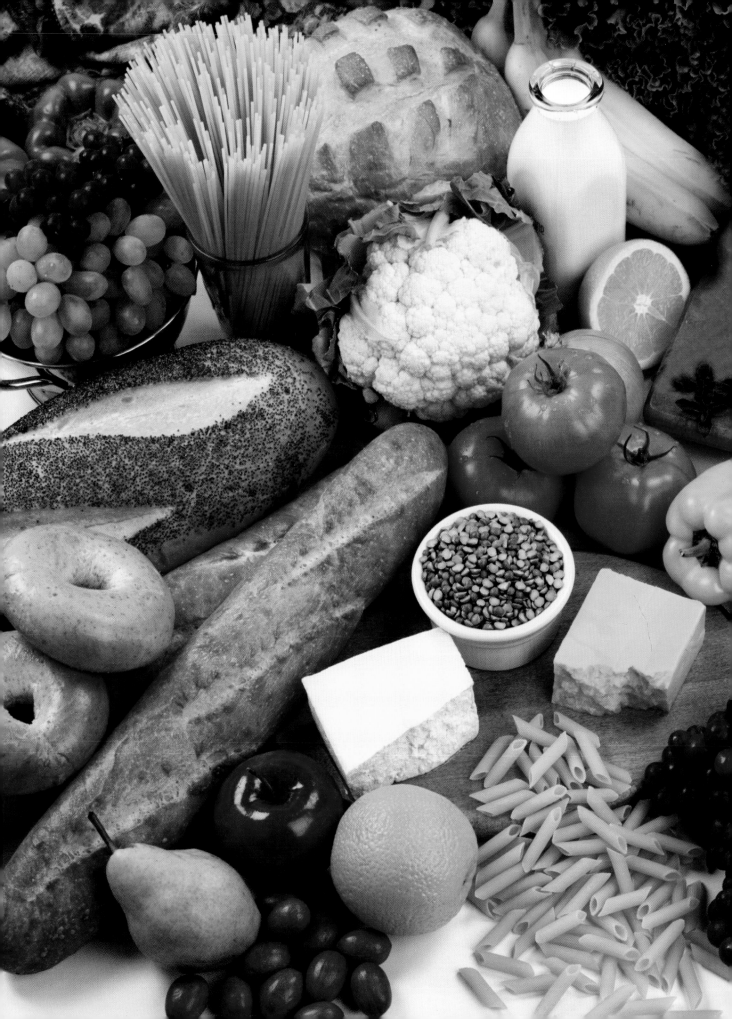

ASANAS

Asanas create a stability in the physical body which then acts as a foundation for the stability of the mind.

These were never meant to be gymnastic skills. Their inspiration came from nature, myth and famous people, so they are named after animals, plants, philosophers and heroes.

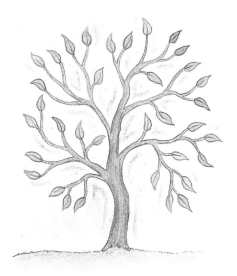

A show of expertise and a polished performance is not the measure of the benefit of each asana. Even incomplete attempts at a position will bring benefits to the nerves, glands and muscles. Traditional texts state that asanas should not be performed by pushing the body past its limits because of the ambitions of the mind.

Asanas are an exploration of the functioning of the physical body so it can become a vehicle for spiritual growth.

They are sometimes known collectively as "Hatha yoga". Here the meaning of "Ha" is the Sun, and "Tha" is the Moon. Hatha, then, describes movements where

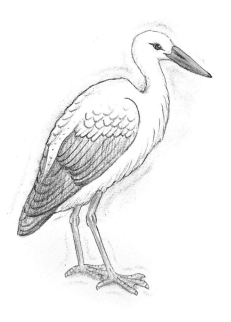

there is a balance of opposites. Each asana features areas of the body where there is rigidity or tension, complemented by areas that are relaxed.

A series of 14 asanas are included here starting on p. 39 and the series known as "Salute to the Sun", on p.78-80.

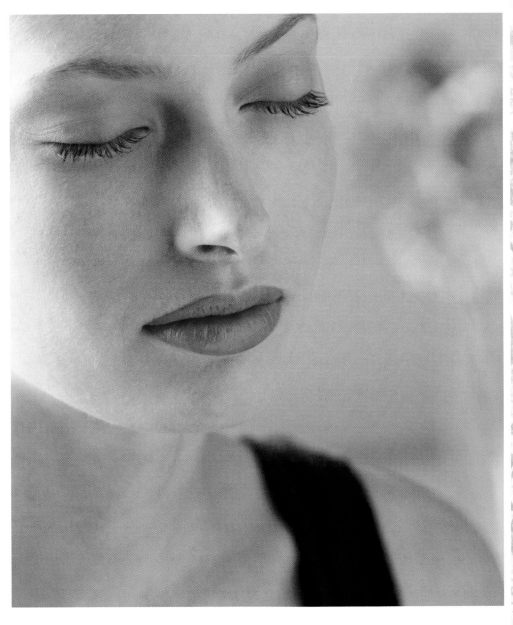

Left: The control and redirection of Pranayama is achieved by harnessing inhalation and exhalation: holding the breath either in or out.

PRANAYAMA

Pranayama is a combination of two words: prana – meaning breath, life-force, energy or chi, and ayama – meaning length, control or stretching.

Pranayama covers a series of breathing techniques that control and redirect the life-force around the body and the nadis. This control and redirection is achieved by harnessing inhalation and exhalation: holding the breath either in or out.

Surya Bhedana (the Sun Breath), Nadi Sodhana (Alternate Nostril Breathing) and Bhamari (the Bee Breath) are covered on p.34-38.

PRATYAHARA

Often referred to as "sense withdrawal" or "sense control", this part of the eight-fold path comes after mastery of the previous four and aims to transform the individual predilections for behaving in certain ways. Pratyahara deals with the understanding of how our mind works so that we can begin to comprehend and then weed out tendencies that will inhibit spiritual growth.

The response of our senses tends to be addictive and so we need to understand how we, as individuals, are caught up in our thoughts and the sensory input that surrounds us. Pratyahara teaches us who is the master and who is the slave; it clarifies who is in charge in our realms of thought as well as in our emotional and habitual behaviour.

The aim is gradually to remove from our lives those activities and beliefs that trap us and tempt us away from where we know we should be.

Traditional texts describe three qualities that permeate the universe:

Sattva – *clarity, purity*
Rajas – *activity, mobility*
Tamas – *inertia, delusion*

The more of the qualities of "sattva" we can achieve, the easier the pathway becomes.

DHARANA

Dharana concerns the functioning of the mind in the preparation for meditation.

It is natural for the mind to be in constant movement. However, the activity of thought needs to be carefully guided to focus at a point where the mind can concentrate on a specific task.

If we sit quietly and observe the mind at work, it becomes clear that it follows lines of thought, one after the other without cease. It is even possible to have two or more trains of thought going on simultaneously. Understanding the nature of the mind in this way helps us to realise how we can work with, rather than against, this natural flow.

The traditional technique for quietening the mind is the repetition of mantra. Mantra is a technique where the meditator repeats words out aloud, whispering or silently in their head, that have a quietening effect on the body and mind (dealt with on p.82-93).

DHYANA AND SAMADHI

These two aspects are translated as meditation and union. They are the natural fruits of all the preceding practices. They are the culmination of this progression and the only way to approach them is to do the practice.

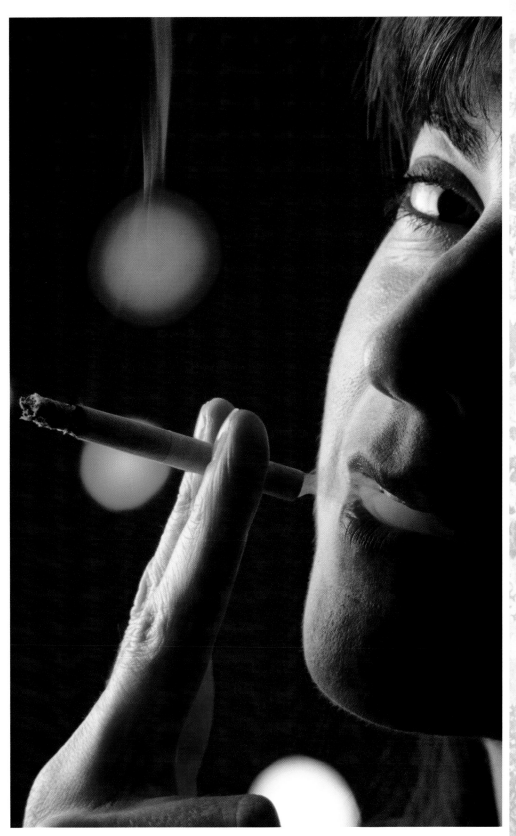

Left: Pratyahara teaches us who is the master and who is the slave; it clarifies who is in charge in our realms of thought as well as in our emotional and habitual behaviour.

GETTING STARTED – THE WESTERN WAY

"Our classes start off with some deep breathing exercises, followed by some general stretching. Next come the postures with their weird names (that's just the English!). At the end of that section, maybe we do some more breathing exercises. Then, "heaven" – the relaxation on the floor where I often drop off to sleep for a while. Then it's back home to raid the fridge, or some weeks we even go into the local café or pub for a drink!"

L.R.S. 1985

Right: a yoga class can be the beginning of a better way of living but in order to gain the full benefits it must find its way into our everyday life.

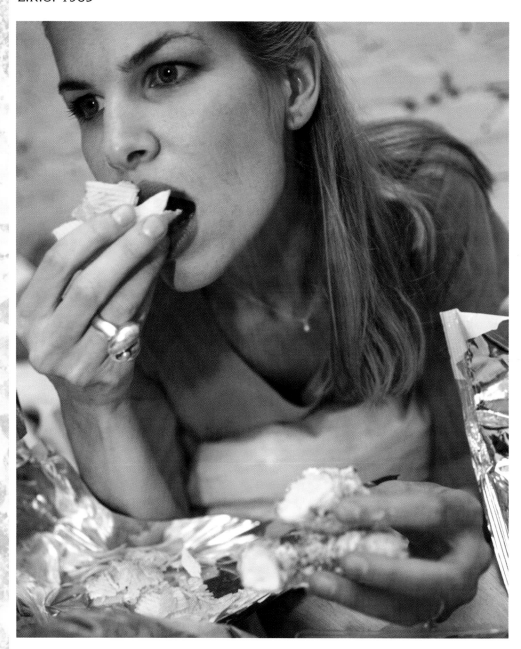

The eight-fold path for most Westerners looks to be a daunting set of steps that seem to have little relevance to how the world works today. In reality, though, it relates exactly to how the world works, but because of expectations, upbringing and dysfunctions now inbuilt into 21st-century society, all may not be apparent.

What tends to attract many people to yoga is the need to relax, to find a gentle way to keep flexible and fit and to feel "better".

For some yoga purists, this all seems to miss the point. However, no matter what attracts us to yoga, if we persist in gentle practice with a balance between breathing, relaxation and good posture work (asanas that are not gymnastic and take account of personal limits), the core of the philosophy manages somehow to find a way into our everyday life.

Babies know how to relax and breathe. They have very flexible joints and they breathe in by relaxing and pushing out their abdomens. By the time most of us are of school age, this inherent flexibility and healthy breathing has disappeared. At 16, our posture is poor, our breathing even worse and we may be recognising that we have a problem relaxing. Unless something is done to alter this situation, by the time we are in our mid-twenties physical symptoms can start to appear.

Eventually stresses will be such that we need to seek medical help to alleviate the various health problems we have accumulated. If we are lucky, this may ease the situation, but in many cases relief will be only temporary. The cycle will continue until eventually orthodox help has no more answers. At this point some sort of self-help may be suggested, and one possibility is yoga.

Most of us arrive at yoga class expecting it to unravel the problems accumulated since childhood ... and sure enough it CAN – though not as rapidly as we might wish.

So let's start with the basics:

Below: babies know how to relax, breathe and have very flexible joints. By the time most of us are of school age, this inherent flexibility and healthy breathing has disappeared.

BREATHING

Most people breathe really badly. They use very little of their full lung capacity. Even divers and athletes may not make the best use of their breath.

There are three levels of breathing:

1 Clavicular Breathing – this is a shallow breath, using only the top part of the lungs, often made worse by breathing in through the mouth. This results in only a small amount of oxygen being breathed in and an equally small amount of carbon dioxide and water vapour being breathed out. This type of breathing contributes to low energy and vitality. People breathing like this may have chronic health problems.

2 Intercostal Breathing – this uses a little more of the lung capacity because the ribcage expands to increase the volume of air taken in.

3 Abdominal Breathing – this is the breathing which babies do and which we all need to practise. It often feels very strange when you first try this sort of breathing. The style is accomplished by the lower abdomen being pushed outwards so that air is drawn in to fill the whole of the lungs. When you breathe out the abdomen is pulled in towards the spine and the diaphragm (the large muscle across the midriff, above your digestive organs, but below your lungs) moves up. This breathing is almost opposite to the "chest out/chin in posture".

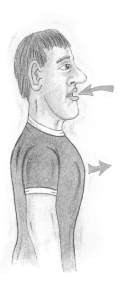
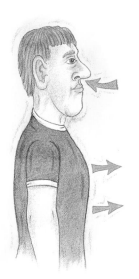
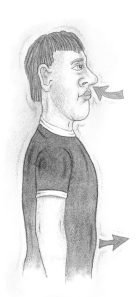

All breathing should be carried out through the nose. This allows the air to be warmed slightly and filters out dust and airborne pollution before the air enters the lungs. The movement of air over the back of the nasal passages is also calming and energising.

Yoga puts emphasis on the exhalation as well as the inhalation. To get good, fresh air in, you need to first breathe out the stale air and excess water vapour from your lungs.

TIPS

If you find this very difficult, do the exercise lying down. Place the palms of your hands on the lower part of the ribs with middle fingers touching. As you breathe in you should feel your hands move apart.

SIMPLE BREATHING EXERCISE

1 *Sit in a position that is comfortable for you, anywhere so long as your back is straight.*

2 *Relax your hands into your lap and tuck your chin in slightly.*

3 *Consciously breathe out through your nose.*

4 *As you breathe in through your nose, keep your shoulders relaxed, allow your stomach to push outwards and try to feel the whole of the trunk of the body filling up with air.*

5 *When you breathe out, pull in the muscles of the stomach, still keeping your shoulders relaxed.*

6 *Repeat 5–10 times.*

Below: if you are sitting when carrying out the breathing exercises make sure you are comfortable, but always keep your back straight.

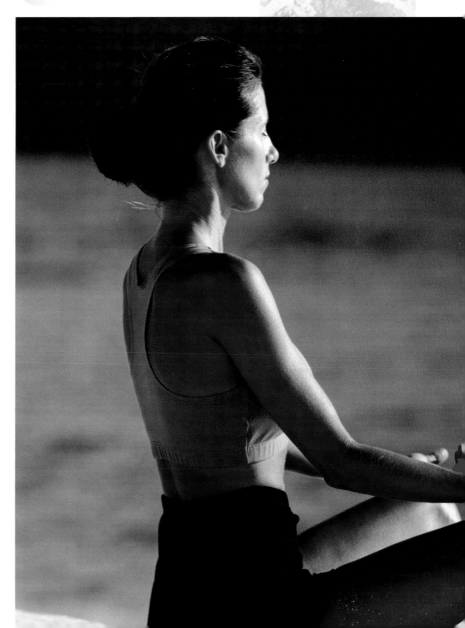

PRANAYAMA

Many of us are aware that when we are scared or excited our breathing speeds up. When we need to concentrate, our breathing slows down. The meaning of pranayama comes from two Sanskrit words – prana, meaning energy or life-force, and yama, meaning restraint or control.

The practice of pranayama regulates and manipulates our breathing to help us to control the state of our mind and thinking processes. It also enables the body to absorb a high level of oxygen from the air.

Of the many traditional pranayamas, here are three with very different properties.

1 – SURYA BHEDANA
Sun Breath

The Sun Breath brings energy into the body and helps the digestion. This pranayama is also very useful in clearing stuffed up noses (have some tissues handy!) and blocked sinuses. It is a great technique to employ if you feel tired or depressed.

1 Sit in a comfortable position with your spine straight, if you are sitting in a chair, try to have your feet touching the floor.

2 Tuck in your chin slightly, so the back of your neck is straight.

3 Rest the back of your left hand on your left knee or thigh, traditionally with thumb and index finger touching.

4 Bring the right hand to the nose.

5 The right thumb, pressing against the right nostril, will act as a valve.

6 The right ring finger on the left nostril also acts like a valve.

7 With the left nostril blocked by the ring finger pressing on the fleshy part, inhale slowly and fully through the right nostril.

8 Close the right nostril with the right thumb.

9 Release the left nostril and breathe out of the left nostril, slowly and fully.

10 This is called "one round of the Sun Breath". This is repeated at least five times.

With practice you may build up to a series of rounds lasting 5–10 minutes.

Don't worry if your breathing sounds like a tyre going down! This is OK.

2 – NADI SODHANA
Alternate Nostril Breathing

This also uses the thumb and ring finger as control valves on the nostrils.

It starts the same way as the Sun Breath.

1 Sit in a comfortable position with your spine straight, if sat in a chair, try to have your feet touching the floor.

2 Tuck in your chin slightly, so the back of your neck is straight.

3 Rest the back of your left hand on your left knee or thigh, traditionally with thumb and index finger touching.

4 Bring the right hand to the nose.

5 The right thumb, pressing against the right nostril, acts as a valve.

6 The right ring finger on the left nostril also acts like a valve.

7 With the left nostril blocked with the ring finger pressing on the fleshy part, inhale slowly and fully through the right nostril.

8 Close the right nostril with the right thumb.

9 Release the left nostril and breathe out of the left nostril, slowly and fully.

10 Keep the right thumb on the right nostril.

11 The next inbreath begins by breathing in through the left nostril.

12 At the end of the inbreath, the left nostril is then closed with the ring finger.

13 The right nostril is opened and the breath released slowly out of the right nostril.

14 This is called "one round of Nadi Sodhana".

The whole sequence is then repeated 5–10 times.

Don't worry if you notice each round taking longer and longer. This is OK. Nadi Sodhana or Alternate Nostril Breathing is very calming and an ideal practice to do just before bedtime or if you are very stressed.

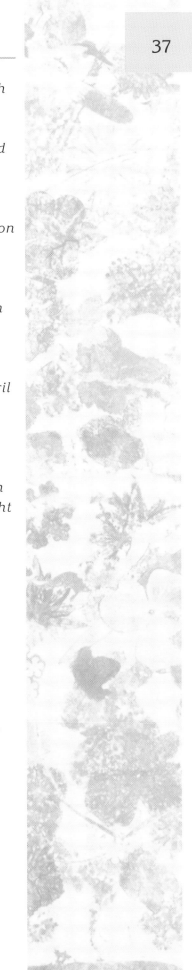

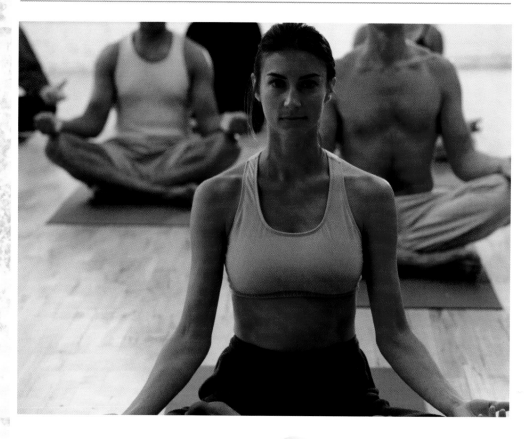

Right: Bee Breath is a good exercise for groups to practise, and becomes a firm favourite once the embarrassment of making a humming sound is overcome.

3 – BRAHMARI
Bee Breath

This is a lovely exercise, excellent help for any breathing problem and good fun to do in groups. Children love to do this exercise.

1 Sit in a comfortable position, with your spine straight.

2 Tuck in your chin.

3 Rest the backs of your hands on your thighs or knees and relax your shoulders.

4 Breathe out slowly and completely.

5 Breathe in.

6 As you breathe out, hum the air out, like a bee, until you have no breath left.

7 You can repeat this. One good "Brahmari" is sometimes sufficient.

Once adults get over the embarrassment of making a noise, this pranayama often becomes a favourite.

Bee Breath is also useful if you have problems sleeping. Expectant mothers find that it can also soothe the baby.

Before you start any of the Hatha yoga postures you need to "set the scene"...

It is a good idea to set aside a room or part of the room especially for your practice.

You will need to sit or lie on a blanket or mat. This will act as a cushion from a hard floor, an anti-slip device when doing standing work and insulation for when you are lying down. Loose clothing is a must – anything that allows you freedom to move and breathe easily is fine.

You should wait an hour or two after a meal before beginning posture work. This allows the body's digestive processes to reach a point where they will not inhibit exercise.

Get yourself focused. Focus on what you are about to do – if you are at home, unplug the phone; resolve not to answer the doorbell; and promise yourself that you will not be rushed.

Sit for a few minutes, breathing deeply or practising one of the pranayamas.

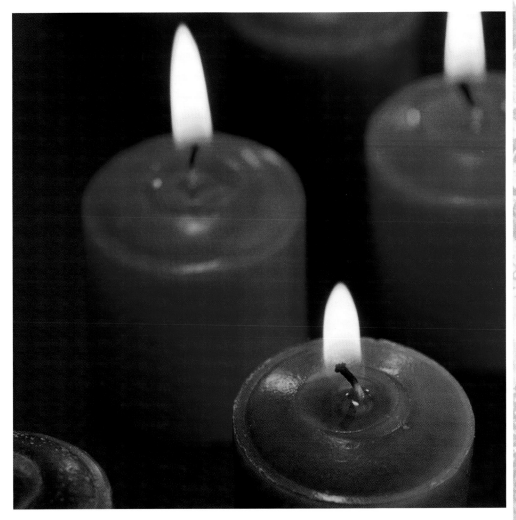

Left: candlelight makes a room with harsh lighting more relaxed and is ideal for "setting the scene".

The following sequence of postures could be used on a daily basis. It is a very gentle sequence with alternatives for use during pregnancy.

POSTURE 1

Stretching (Pavanmuktasana)

This is ideal to do as a warm-up before beginning the postures.

1 Lie flat on the floor, on your blanket or mat.

2 Breathing in, bend your left leg at the knee, clasping your hands around the knee and bring the knee down onto your chest.

3 Breathing out, stretch your leg out straight.

4 Place the palms of your hands on the floor down by your side.

5 Slowly lower the leg to the ground.

6 Repeat the same with the right leg.

7 Repeat the whole sequence 3–5 times.

TIPS

When lowering your legs, press the palms of your hands into the floor. This helps to give a steady rate of descent!

Don't worry if you find yourself passing wind. This exercise massages the digestive system and often releases trapped wind – either end!

REMEMBER:
Postures are not gymnastic exercises. They are designed to help energy to flow more easily around the body, not to develop lots of muscles.

In each posture you try, explore how your body moves (or not!). Pushing yourself past discomfort into pain is not yoga.

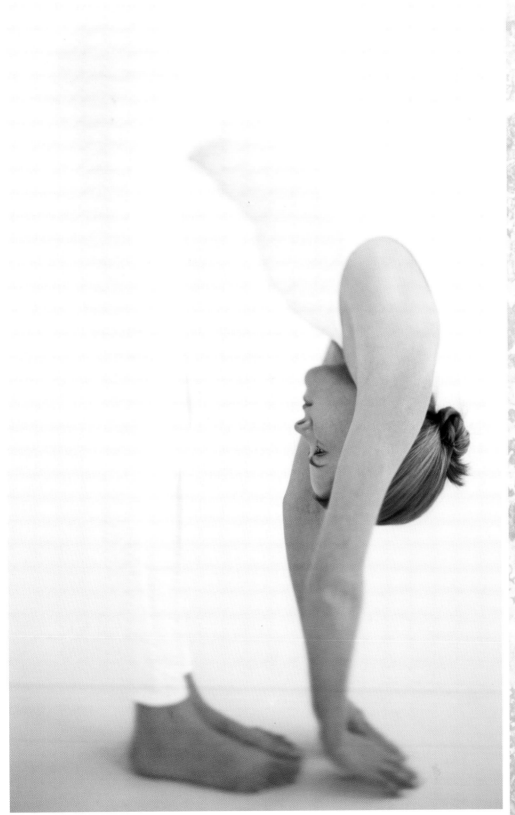

Left: it is important to warm up using gentle stretching exercises before begining yoga.

POSTURE 2 –

Mountain Posture
Tadasana

This may seem a strange one to start with – that is – just "standing up". This posture, though, has its subtleties and can be more difficult than you think.

1 Stand with your feet together. The big toes should be touching each other, the heels apart a little.

2 Try to feel the floor where your feet touch it.

3 Lock your knees.

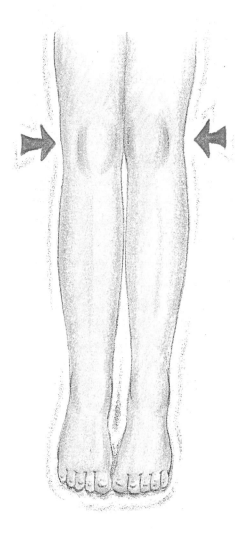

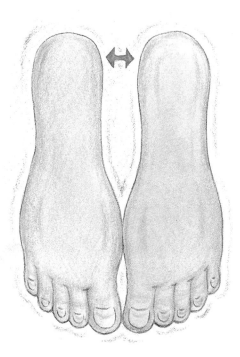

4 Tuck in your bottom.

5 Relax your shoulders, letting your arms hang freely.

6 Tuck in your chin.

7 Relax your gaze to an area about two metres away from you, on the floor.

TIPS

· Imagine the centre of the top of your head being attached to the ceiling by a thread.

· Make sure your weight is evenly balanced from the front to the back of your feet, as well as evenly on the right and left.

· Remember to breathe normally!

· Don't worry if you find yourself swaying or wobbling a bit. Just re-focus your gaze on the floor about two metres in front of you.

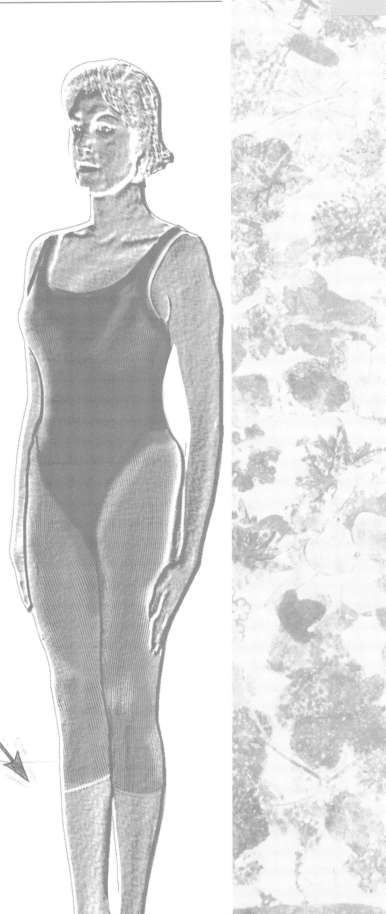

POSTURE 3

Hands-to-Feet
Padangusthasana

1 *Stand in the Mountain Posture (Tadasana).*

2 *Breathe in, raising your arms above your head, fingers extended.*

3 *As you breathe out, bend forward a little, reaching forward with your arms.*

4 *Continue to bend the trunk of your body forward gently until you reach your natural limit.*

TIPS

Reaching forward, before bending forward, helps you to bend at the hips and not at the waist.

Try not to stick your bottom out behind you as you bend forward. Theoretically, this posture could be done with you standing with your back against a wall!

This posture works mainly on the base chakra

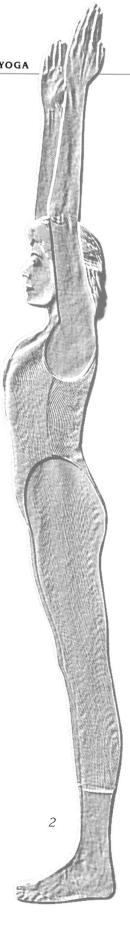

2

5 Bring your arms to rest comfortably on your legs.

6 Lower your head and relax your neck and back muscles; the leg muscles stay strong.

7 Breathe normally.

8 When you are ready to come up, breathe in and slowly uncurl your back, into its upright position.

9 Breathe out.

TIPS

When and if your hands and fingers do make contact with your feet, wrap your fingers around each big toe.

Don't worry if your hands don't reach your feet – it may be quite a while until your back is relaxed enough to allow this to happen.

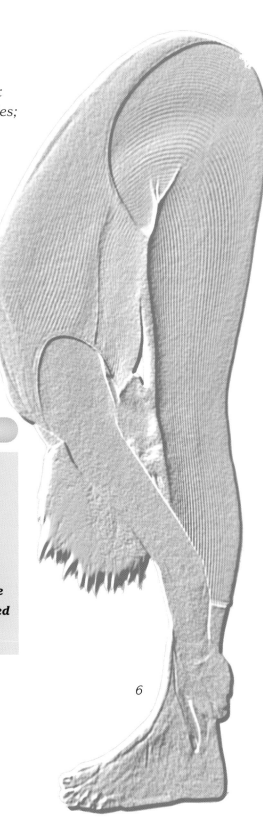

6

POSTURE 4
The Warrior –
Virhabhadrasana

1 Stand in the Mountain
Posture (Tadasana).

2 Move your feet apart. The
ideal distance is five of your
foot-lengths, but do what you
can manage. This distance
creates certain energy dynamics
in the muscles and tendons, and
also helps to reproduce these
each time you do the posture.

*Below: a group
performing 'The
Warrior' at step '5'.*

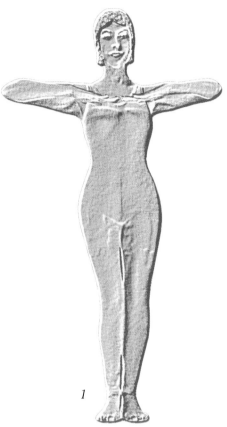

1

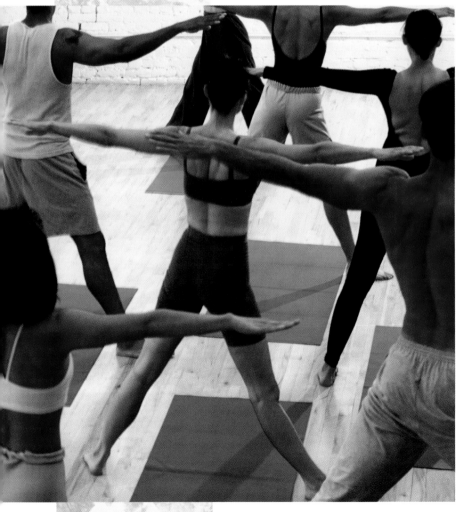

3 Begin by focusing on your
left, by turning the left foot,
a quarter turn, anticlockwise.

4 Turn the right foot slightly
anticlockwise.

5 Breathe in, bringing your
arms up to shoulder height,
stretching them out to either
side, palms up.

6 As you breathe out, bend
your left knee, and look
down the line of your left arm.

7 Breathe
normally.

This posture works effectively on the base and sacral chakras and creates an increase in the flow of blood all around the body, but particularly in the legs.

8 When you are ready to come out of the posture, breathe in, straighten your left leg and move your feet around to face the front.

9 Repeat, mirroring the above movement on the right side.

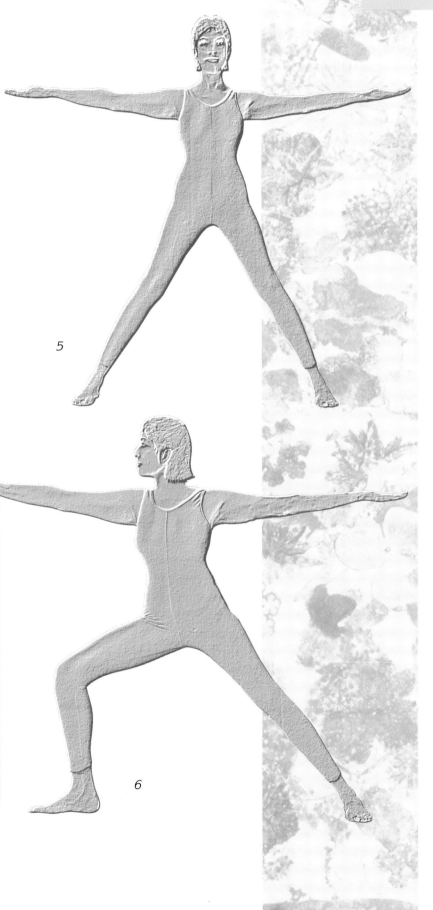

5

6

TIPS

Virhabhadra was a very proud warrior so this pose should convey that sort of feeling. It is very strong.

When you are practised in this asana, it should appear to an onlooker that you are sat on an invisible chair and have an invisible box under the bent leg.

Don't worry if you seem to get nowhere with this one at first. If you find it difficult to hold the "invisible chair" part of the posture, you can lean slightly to the side where the leg is bent. Gradually straighten the spine as you become stronger.

POSTURE 5
Triangle
Trikonasana

Trikonasana works on the solar plexus chakra.

1 Stand in the Mountain Posture (Tadasana).

2 Move your feet apart. The ideal distance is three and a half of your foot-lengths. Like the Warrior Posture this is fairly precise and creates specific activity in certain muscles and tendons.

3 Begin by focusing on the left by turning the left foot a quarter turn outwards (anticlockwise).

4 Turn the right foot anticlockwise very slightly.

5 Bring your arms up to shoulder height, stretched out to each side.

6 Stretch outwards to the left and begin to swing your left arm down and the right arm up.

7 As you stretch your arm down to the left, tilt your left hip downwards and your right hip upwards.

8 Tilt the whole of your body sideways to the left, until you reach your natural limit.

9 Then allow your arms to continue the swing until your left hand makes contact with your left leg.

10 Allow your right arm to continue until it is vertical.

5

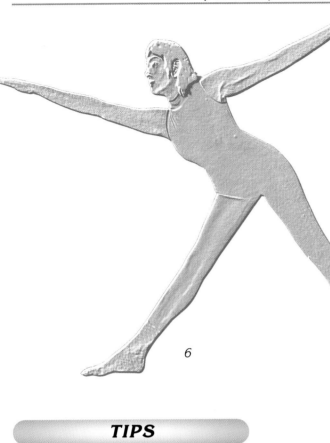

6

10

TIPS

This posture is excellent for toning up the waist and hips. Traditionally, you would do this posture starting with your back against a wall. This is a good idea while you are getting used to the posture. It helps to stop the tendency to bend forward as you stretch down to either side.

Don't worry if, when you begin to try this posture, you find you don't move very far. It is dependent on the flexibility of the lower back and stretching out of the ribcage. This develops as you practise the posture regularly.

11 Breathe normally.

12 When you are ready to come out of the posture, breathe in and bring the trunk of your body back to vertical.

13 Move your feet back to the front.

14 Repeat, mirroring the movement down to the right.

Right: the Reversed or Twisted Triangle being practised in a group.

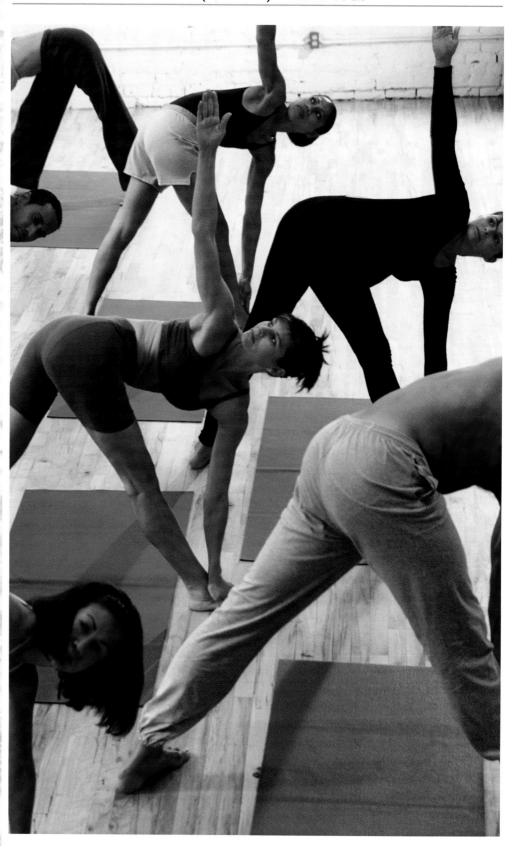

POSTURE **6**

Face of a Cow
Gumukhasana

1 Kneel on your blanket or mat, sitting back on your heels. If this is uncomfortable, you can roll another blanket placing it between your legs to support your bottom. You can also do this posture sat on a stool.

2 Stretch both arms out in front of you.

3 Raise your left arm over your head, bending at the elbow so that the left hand rests near the top of your back.

4 Sweep your right arm around to the right side, bending at the elbow, sending the right hand up the back.

5 If your hands meet, lightly clasp your fingers.

6 If your hands do not meet, repeat steps 1–4, holding one end of a piece of cane or dowling about 25–30 cms long in the left hand. You should then be able to clasp the other end of the cane with your right hand.

7 When you have a grip, take a breath in and bring your fingers/hands closer together.

8 On the outbreath, slowly bend forward until you reach your natural limit.

9 Breathe naturally.

10 When you are ready to come out of the posture, breathe in and sit up.

11 Loosen your grip and repeat, mirroring the above stages, starting with raising the right hand above the head.

TIPS

This posture helps to expand the chest and loosen the shoulders. Don't worry if you get virtually nowhere when you first try this one! It releases tension in the shoulders and neck so effectively, you will be surprised how quickly you can become proficient.

This posture works on the heart chakra.

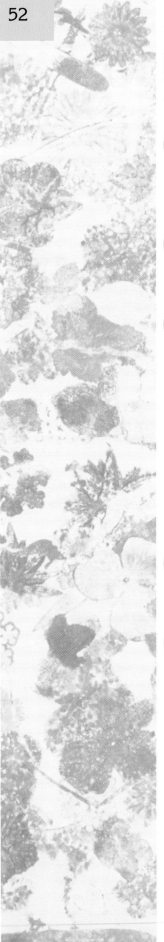

POSTURE 7
Fish
Matsyasana

1 *Begin by sitting on your blanket or mat with your legs out in front of you and your feet together.*

2 *Place the palms of your hands on both hips, bending your elbows behind you.*

3 *Lean back onto your elbows and breathe in.*

4

4 *As you breathe out, allow the head to drop backwards and arch your back slightly.*

5 *Breathe normally.*

6

6 *When you want to come out of the posture, allow your elbows to slide away, lowering yourself into a lying position.*

7 Roll onto one side and sit up from there.

TIPS

This posture helps to improve breathing and the healthy activity of the thyroid. It can be useful when poor breathing techniques or thyroid difficulties are aggravating excess weight.

Don't worry if you feel pressure on your throat when you first do this posture – this gives an indication that you will benefit from it. If it is very uncomfortable, only do it for very short periods.

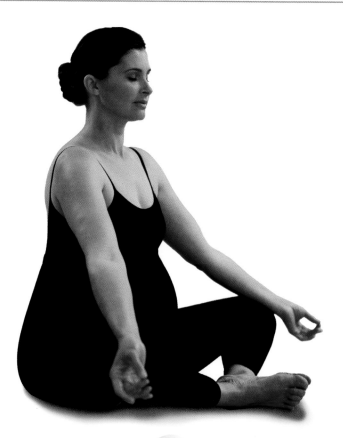

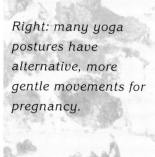

Right: many yoga postures have alternative, more gentle movements for pregnancy.

Please note – alternative posture for pregnancy: a very gentle version of Ustrasana (the Camel Posture)

Unless you are used to the Fish Posture it would be a good idea to adopt this gentle version of the Camel Posture (Ustrasana) if you are more than 12 weeks into pregnancy.

1 On your blanket or mat adopt the posture of sitting on your heels, using a rolled-up blanket under you if you find this uncomfortable.

2 Clasp your hands behind you.

3 Breathe in and, as you breathe out, allow your neck to drop backwards. At the same time, raise your arms a little behind you.

4 Breathe normally.

5 When you are ready to come out of the posture, bring yourself back to sitting straight on an outbreath.

Both of these postures work on the throat and brow chakras.

POSTURE 8
Dog
Adho Mukha Svanasana

1 *Kneel on your blanket or mat on all fours, making sure your knees are in a straight line under your hips.*

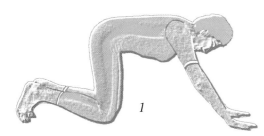

1

2 *Make sure that your hands are directly under your shoulders and spread your fingers.*

3 *Tuck your toes under, so they are in contact with your blanket or mat.*

4 *Breathe in, lifting your pelvis and straightening your legs, keeping your head low.*

4

5 *Allow your heels to relax downwards, towards the floor.*

TIPS

• *As you do this posture imagine your bottom is lifting up towards the ceiling and you are stretching your back like a dog or cat does when it first wakes.*

• *Don't worry if you find yourself noticing any pressure in the head – gently bring yourself out of the posture. This will diminish as you practise.*

6 *Breathe naturally.*

7 *Stay in the posture until you feel you have reached your natural limit.*

8 *Breathe in and, as you breathe out, lower yourself back onto all fours.*

9 *Slide yourself back until you are sitting on your heels, rest your forehead on the floor and relax.*

This posture works on the brow and crown chakras.

9

POSTURE 9
Cobra
Bhujangasana

1 *Lie flat on your blanket or mat, face downwards.*

2 *Breathe in, placing the hands, palms down, under the chest.*

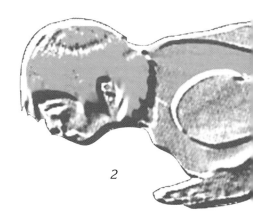

2

4 *As you breathe in, gently raise the top part of your body a little. If you feel pressure in the middle of your back – don't go any higher.*

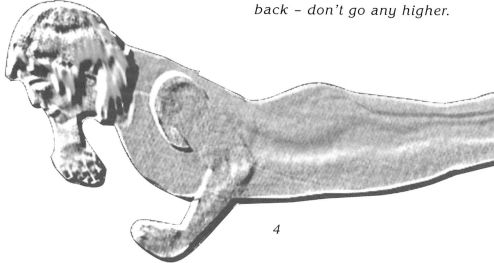

4

3 *Breathe out, checking that your toes are relaxed and the tops of your feet are flat on the floor.*

Bhujangasana works on opening up the chest and heart chakra and stretches the spine.

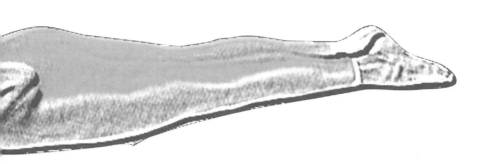

5 Hold the posture, breathing naturally, looking straight ahead.

6 When you are ready to release the posture, breathe in and, as you breathe out, lower yourself back to the floor.

TIPS

If you tighten the muscles in your buttocks when you lift the torso, you will lift in the correct way. This posture is not a back bend; it is a lift from the pelvis. Don't worry if you only lift a little. It is better to lift the body a little and correctly than a lot and badly.

Please note: if you are further than 12 weeks into a pregnancy, you may find this one uncomfortable. You can repeat Gumukhasana (Face of a Cow) at this point in the sequence.

5

POSTURE 10
Spinal Twist
Matsyendrasana

1 Kneel down on your blanket or mat, resting on your heels.

2 Slide your buttocks to the right of your feet.

3 Lift your left leg, so the left foot is over the right knee.

4 Shuffle your bottom around to get comfortable and to keep your spine straight.

5 Bring your left arm round behind you to the left, resting your fingers on the floor to steady yourself.

6 Bring your right arm to rest on the outside of your left leg, the elbow bracing against the knee.

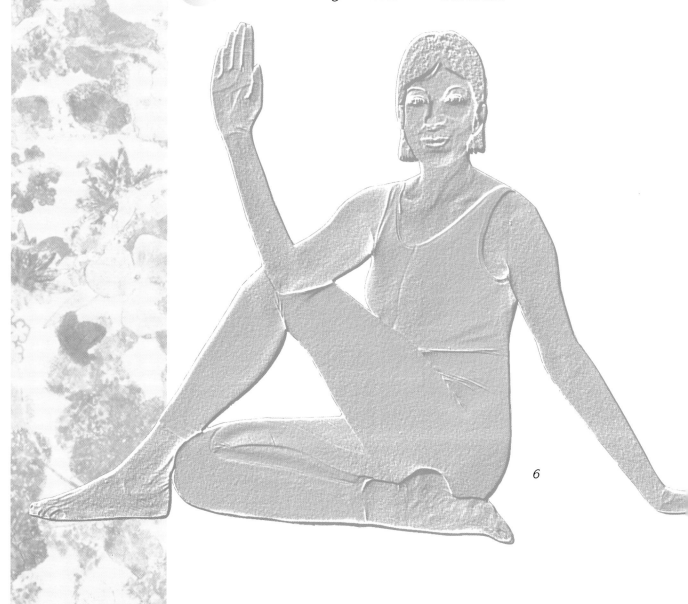

6

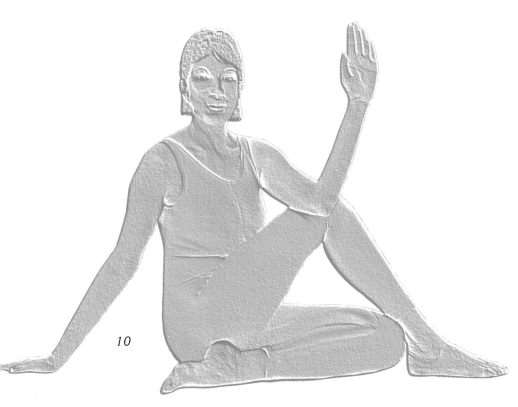

10

7 Breathe in and, as you breathe out, lift your spine and twist round to look over your left shoulder.

8 Breathe normally.

9 When you are ready to release the pose, breathe in and, as you breathe out, unwind yourself.

10 Repeat, mirroring the steps, starting with sliding your seat to the left of your feet.

This posture works on the solar plexus chakra, the sacral chakra and the whole of the spine.

TIPS

The more upright you can keep your spine, the easier it is to twist.

If you are well padded in the midriff, lifting the spine also helps to create the space to twist.

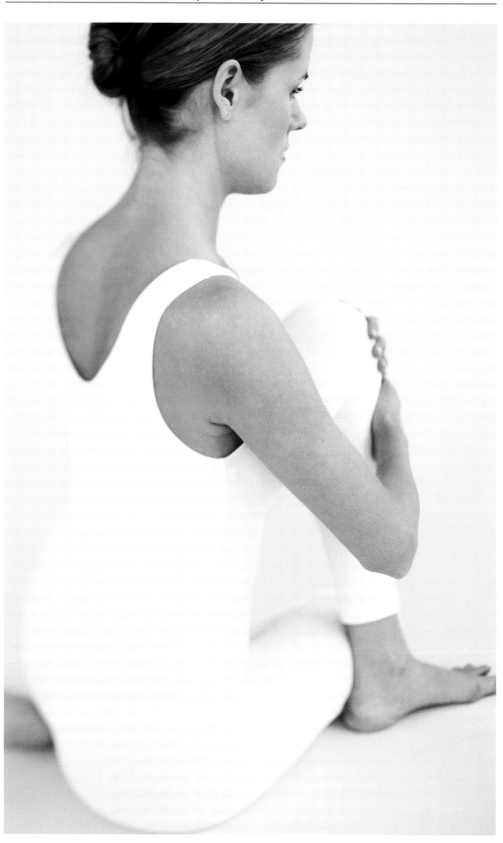

Right: when doing the 'Spinal Twist' remember to keep your spine vertical.

POSTURE 11

Forward Bend
Paschimottanasana

1 Sit on your blanket or mat, with your legs stretched out in front of you.

2 As you breathe in, lift your arms above your head, stretching your ribcage.

3 As you breathe out, lower your arms, reaching out for the floor beyond your feet.

4 When you have reached your natural limit of bending forward, relax your arms, letting your hands relax onto your legs/ankles/feet – whichever is comfortable.

5 Breathe naturally.

6 On each inbreath, lift your body up a little, stretching your back.

7 On each outbreath, relax your neck, shoulders, arms and hands.

8 Continue breathing, stretching and relaxing in this fashion until you are ready to come out of the posture.

9 On an inbreath, bring yourself back up to sitting.

This posture works on the sacral and base chakras.

TIPS

When you initially sit on your blanket or mat, make sure you are sitting on your "sit" bones.

These are the ones that dig into the blanket or mat. If you are well-padded here, ease some of your padding away to the side to allow better contact of your "sit" bones with the floor.

The hip joints are the pivot for this posture; bending at the waist is not correct.

Don't worry if you find you hardly bend forward at all. If you follow the steps here, you will find this happening naturally with practice. Grabbing hold of your knees/calves/ankles and pulling will only damage ligaments and tendons. The breath is sufficient focus.

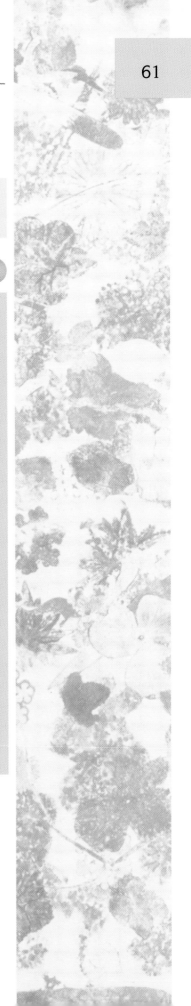

POSTURE 12
Easy Posture
Mukasana

1 *Sit on your blanket or mat with your legs out in front of you, slightly apart.*

2 *Bend your right leg and bring your right foot in towards your pubic bone.*

3 *Tuck the right heel against the pubic bone, so the top of the foot lies on the floor.*

4 *Bend your left leg and bring your left foot to lie alongside the right, the heels in line with each other.*

5 *On an inbreath, straighten your spine and relax your shoulders.*

6 *Breathe naturally.*

7 *Repeat, with the left foot against the pubic bone first.*

This posture is part of a series that prepares the body to sit in the Lotus Posture (Padmasana) The Easy Posture works on the base chakra.

TIPS

You may find it easier at first, if you slip a small cushion just under the buttocks or the base of the spine.

Don't worry if your knees or lower legs don't touch the floor. The more you relax into this posture, the more comfortable you will feel and the more flexible your legs will become.

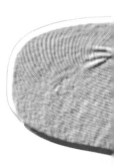

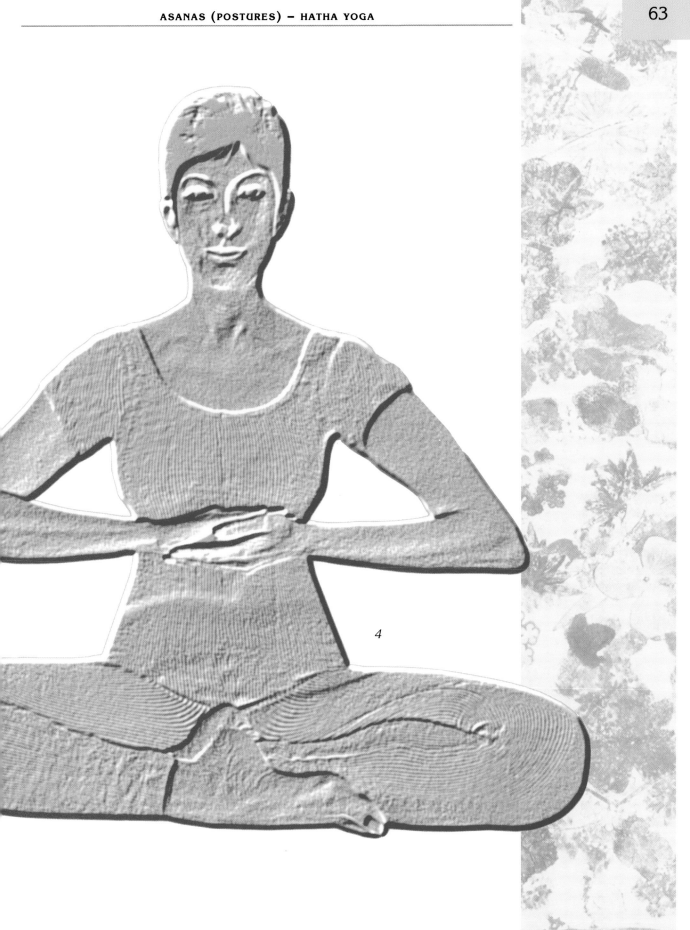

4

POSTURE 13
The Cobbler's Posture
Baddha Konasana

1 Sit on your blanket or mat, with your legs stretched out in front of you.

2 Bend both knees, bringing your feet nearer your body.

3 Bring the soles of the feet together, holding your feet, and pulling the heels towards your pubic bone.

4 As you breathe in, straighten your spine.

5 As you breathe out, relax your legs.

3

TIPS

The key to this posture is relaxation of the tendons on the inside of the thighs.

Do NOT force your knees down to the floor. You can rest your wrists on your knees – that is all!

Don't worry if it takes ages before you see any improvement in the relaxation of your legs so that they rest on the floor.

This is an excellent posture to practise whilst doing other tasks outside of your yoga session. Small children and some adults find this posture very easy – try not to get too disheartened!

This posture works on the base chakra but also has a terrific healing effect on the reproductive organs for men and women. This is an ideal posture to help with menstrual difficulties, sciatica and hernias. It is renowned for refreshing the blood supply to the pelvis, lower abdomen, kidneys and bladder. Excellent for enhancing your sex life!

6 Continue with this breathing cycle, until you are ready to leave the posture.

4

7 Breathe in and, as you breathe out, release your legs, returning them to straight in front of you.

POSTURE **14**

Corpse Posture
Savasana

1 Lie flat on your back on your blanket or mat.

2 Rest you hands a little away from your body, palms up.

3 Your feet may be more comfortable if they are apart a little. Allow them to relax.

4 Stretch your feet away from you, to lengthen your legs, and then relax.

TIPS

You need to be warm to relax. On very cold days you may need an extra blanket underneath you, as well as one wrapped around you.

   Don't worry if you fall asleep! It may take a while to stay conscious for a full 20 minutes.

5 Try to spread your shoulders so that as much of the top of your back and neck touches the floor as you can manage.

6 Tuck in your chin.

7 Close your eyes.

8 Take a deep breath in and, as you breathe out, allow yourself to sink into the floor.

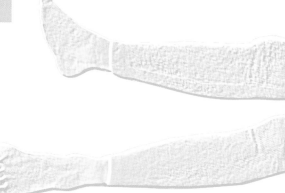

9 *Continue being aware of your breathing, but without strain, for 5–20 minutes.*

If the weather is cool, make sure you have a blanket or cover for yourself for this posture.

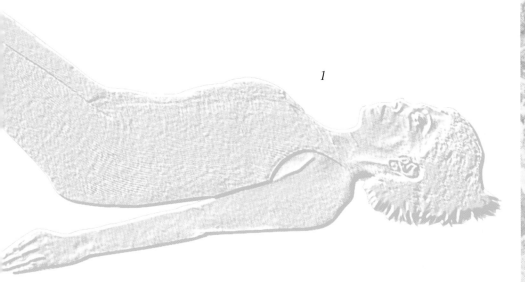

1

The more you are able to relax, the more prana/energy/chi flows around your body. This enables the body to refresh and heal itself.

You may wish to include one of the relaxation techniques from the next chapter as part of Savasana.

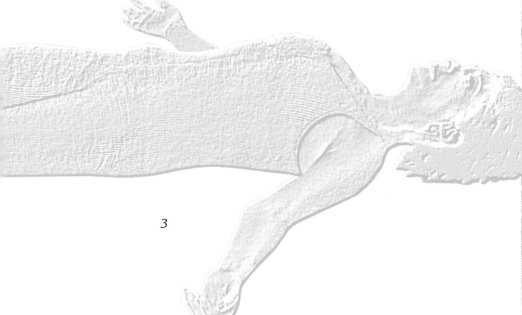

3

RELAXATION

From a therapeutic point of view, the need to relax is probably the most common reason that people in the West are drawn to yoga. Relaxation often has to be completely relearned once levels of stress or hyperactivity begin to take a toll on physical or emotional health.

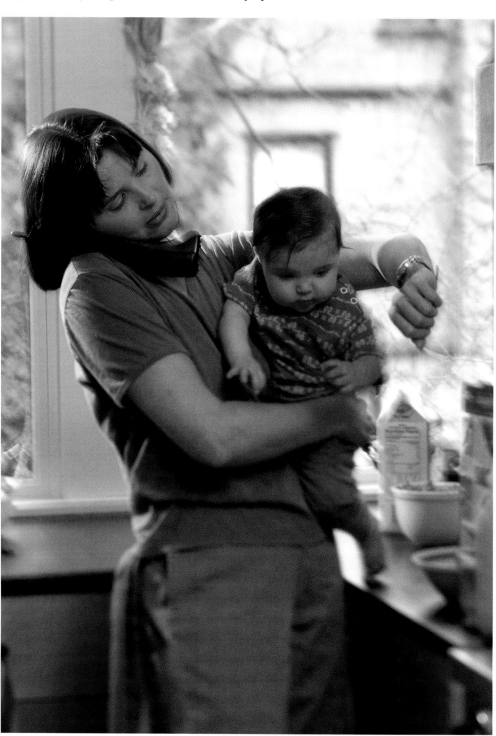

Right: the need to relax is probably the most common reason that people in the West are drawn to yoga.

The following relaxation techniques can be recorded onto a tape for you to use if you wish. Listening to a voice talking you through relaxation is often more effective than taking yourself mentally through the procedure.

The easiest posture to adopt for relaxation is the Corpse Posture (Savasana), but you can do this sat somewhere where you feel comfortable.

Considerations:

1. If you have back or other muscle problems, you may find placing a cushion under your knees and/or a small cushion under your neck, more comfortable.

2. You may prefer to have an extra blanket to keep yourself warm, as the body temperature often lowers during relaxation.

3. Set aside a specific time. Turn off the phone and the radio and resolve to ignore potential disruptions.

Begin each session with a few minutes of deep breathing, or a pranayama.

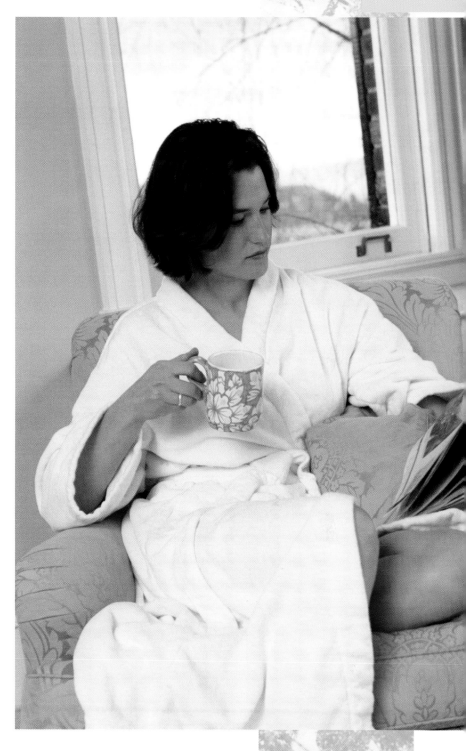

Above: find time to relax and ignore potential disruptions.

RELAXATION 1

1 Lie on your blanket or mat in the Corpse Posture (Savasana) and close your eyes.

2 On an outbreath, allow your body to sink into the floor.

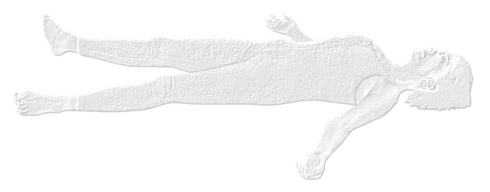

3 Point your toes away from you, tensing the muscles of your legs. Hold for the count of ten, and then release.

4 Clench your fists, pushing them away from your body, tensing the muscles in your arms, hold for a count of ten, and then relax.

5 Tuck in your chin, stretching the back of the neck, and relax.

6 Swallow and allow your jaw to drop slightly, releasing the muscles.

7 Switch your attention to your breathing.

8 Without controlling the breath in any way, allow yourself to sink further into the floor a little more on each outbreath.

9 Continue for between five and 20 minutes.

10 When you are ready to come out of the relaxation, stretch your feet and move your hands.

11 Turn onto your side to bring yourself to sitting.

TIPS

Start off with five minutes if you are not used to relaxation techniques. Build up to 20 over a period of several weeks of daily practice.

You may want to set a clock alarm initially, to ensure you stay in the relaxation for at least five minutes!

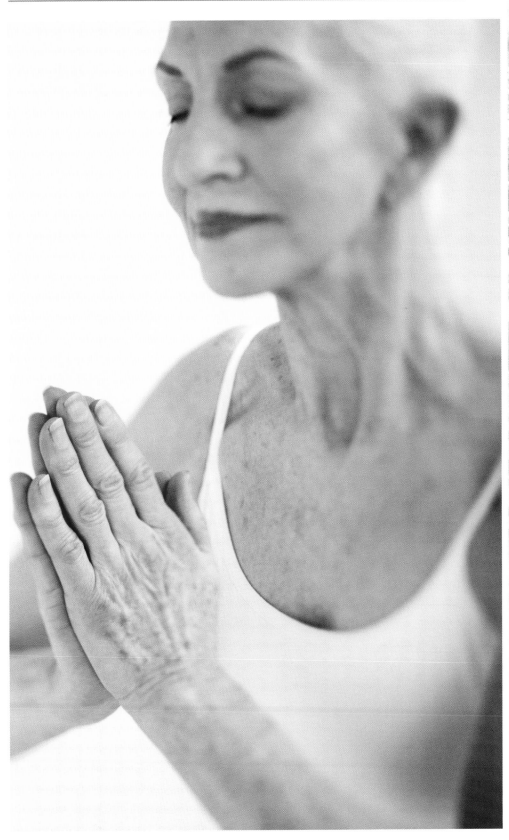

*Left: relaxation can
take on many forms
including the deep
relaxation achieved
when meditating.*

RELAXATION 2

1 Lie on your blanket or mat in the Corpse Posture (Savasana) and close your eyes.

2 On an outbreath, allow your body to sink into the floor.

3 Point your toes away from you, tensing the muscles of the legs. Hold for the count of ten, and then release.

4 Clench your fists, pushing them away from your body, tensing the muscles in your arms, hold for a count of ten, and then relax.

5 Tuck in your chin, stretching the back of the neck, and relax.

6 Swallow and allow your jaw to drop slightly, releasing the muscles.

3

4

7 Switch your attention to the following parts of the body.

Do not actually move them, just mentally "touch" them. They need to come in quick succession.

Right big toe, second toe, third toe, fourth toe, fifth toe
... ball of the foot, instep, top of the foot, heel.
... Lower leg, back of the knee, top of the knee, top of the thigh, back of the thigh, right buttock.
Left big toe, second toe, third toe, fourth toe, fifth toe
... ball of the foot, instep, top of the foot, heel
... lower leg, back of the knee, top of the knee, top of the thigh, back of the thigh, left buttock.
The right side of the back
... the right side from the hip to the armpit, the right side of the chest
... The left side of the back, the left side from the hip to the armpit, the left side of the chest.

The right thumb, first finger, second finger, third finger, fourth finger
... palm of your hand, back of your hand
... the lower arm, elbow, upper arm
... right shoulder.

The left thumb, first finger, second finger, third finger, fourth finger
... palm of your hand, back of your hand
... the lower arm, elbow, upper arm
... left shoulder.
The right eye, the left eye
... the right ear, the left ear
... the right cheek, the left cheek
... the tongue and the muscles inside the mouth.

TIPS

You can "talk through the body" twice if you are particularly stressed – though you might find you go to sleep before the end of the second run.

8 Switch your attention to your breathing, without trying to control the breath.

9 When you are ready to come out of the relaxation, stretch your toes, and move your fingers.

10 Turn onto your side and slowly bring yourself to sitting.

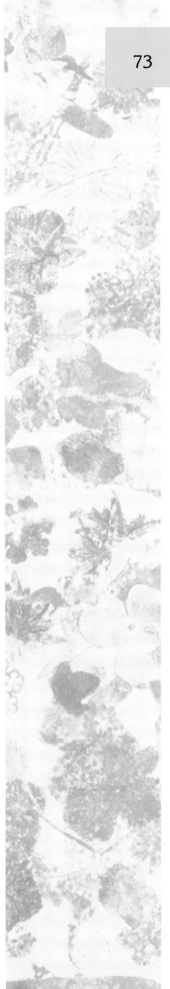

LITTLE YOGA NIDRA/SLEEP

Begin in the same way as
Relaxation 2:

1 Lie on your blanket or mat in the Corpse Posture (Savasana) and close your eyes.

2 On an outbreath, allow your body to sink into the floor.

3 Point your toes away from you, tensing the muscles of the legs. Hold for the count of ten, and then release.

4 Clench your fists, pushing them away from your body, tensing the muscles in your arms, hold for a count of ten, and then relax.

5 Tuck in your chin, stretching the back of the neck, and relax.

6 Swallow and allow your jaw to drop slightly, releasing the muscles.

7 You can, at this point, "talk through the body" as in Relaxation 2, if you wish. If not, go straight to 8.

8 Turn your attention to your ears and listen to every noise in and outside of the room. Keep this up for about 2–3 minutes.

9 Switch your attention to your breathing, and imagine the breath is coming into your body through the soles of your feet. Do this for 3–5 breaths.

10 "Send" the next five outbreaths to the base of the spine

11 The next five outbreaths go to the area below and behind the navel.

12 The next five outbreaths are sent to the area just below the ribcage.

13 The next five go to the centre of the chest.

14 The next five are sent to the throat.

15 The next five outbreaths go to the centre of the forehead.

16 The next five go to the top of the head.

If you are having trouble going to sleep because your mind will not quieten – this technique is very effective.

17 At the next inbreath, imagine the air flowing from your feet, right up to the top of your head.

18 With the next outbreath, imagine the air flowing from the top of your head, right down to your feet.

19 Repeat steps 17 and 18 four more times.

20 Allow the focus of the breath to fade.

21 Rest with your body, without focus, for 2–5 minutes.

22 Gently move your toes and your fingers, and open your eyes.

23 Turn onto your side to bring yourself to sitting, and out of the relaxation.

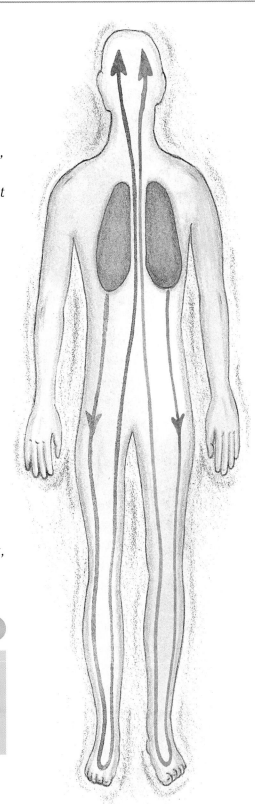

TIPS

If the room you are using for practice is cold, you will need to be well wrapped up and warm to get maximum benefit.

ESTABLISHING A DAILY ROUTINE

It needs to be appreciated that the function of the first two limbs of the traditional eight-fold path were designed to prepare the yoga student for postures, by clearing out the subtle energy channels of the body. Here in the West, we often jump straight into Hatha yoga practice and, unless we take it slowly and with awareness, our bodies and minds may not cope particularly well with the changes yoga creates.

When beginning regular yoga practice it is a good idea to be circumspect and cautious in how you treat your body and not to become extreme in your efforts.

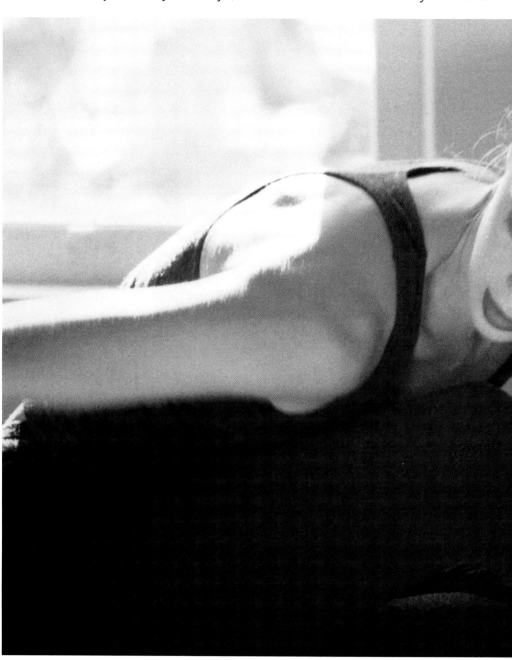

Right: when first practising yoga, do not become too extreme in your efforts, start with a gentle daily routine.

Following the format of "breathing, postures, relaxation" is an excellent place to start. When you become more practised, you can add meditation.

The posture sequence covered in this book is a balanced practice in itself and an excellent one to adopt as a regular routine.

However, there is another traditional set sequence that can be used with, instead of, or as an alternate daily routine.

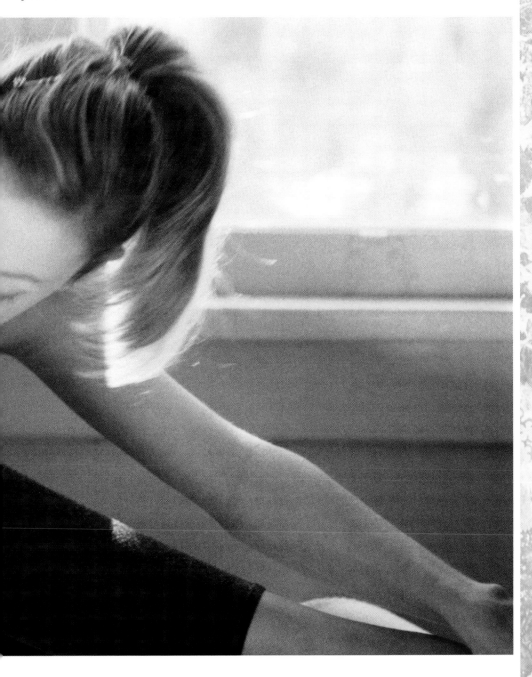

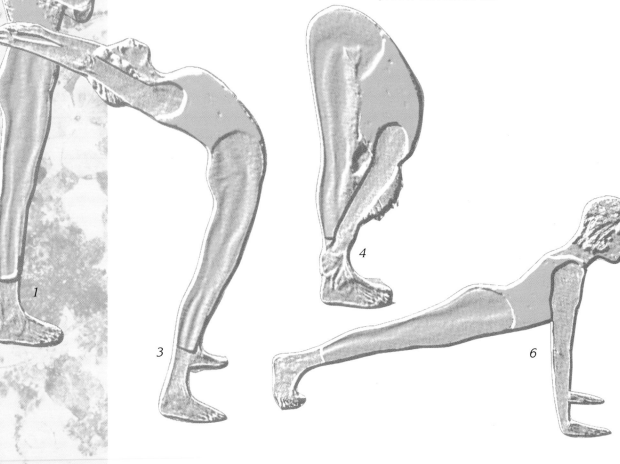

THE SALUTE TO THE SUN
Surya Namaskar

1 Begin by deep breathing or practising pranayama (5–10 minutes).

2 Stand in the Mountain Posture (Tadasana) and bring your palms together in the traditional "prayer" position in front of the centre of your chest. Breathe in and out.

3 On the next inbreath, stretch your arms up above your head and lean back from your waist, looking up towards your hands.

4 On the outbreath, straighten and bend forward from the hips with the intention of reaching the floor with your hands. (Don't worry if you have to bend your knees.) Place your hands on the floor, the finger tips in line with your toes.

5 On the next inbreath, send your right leg back so the knee touches the floor and the toes are tucked under. Look upwards.

6 On the outbreath, lower your head and send your left leg out to join the right leg, behind you. Allow your bottom to lift upwards away from the floor. Breathe in.

1

3

4

6

7 On the next outbreath, lower yourself, bending your knees so they touch the floor, continue lowering the chest to the floor, then your chin. (The hips stay off the floor.)

8 On the next inbreath, lower your hips, flatten your toes and lift your head and chest up, straightening your arms. Look upwards.

9 On the next outbreath, tuck your toes back under and, pressing on your hands, lift your hips so they are the highest part of you off the floor. Lower your head.

10 Breathing in (lifting your chin so your knee doesn't catch it), bring your left foot forwards between your hands. (Don't worry if you have to shuffle your body around a bit to do this.) Look upwards.

11 Breathing out, bring the right foot up to join the left, creating a forward bend. Keep your head low.

12 The next inbreath takes you upright again, leaning back slightly, with your hands above your head. Look upwards.

13 On the outbreath, lower your arms and return to the Mountain Posture (Tadasana).

7

11

8

This is just one round of Salute to the Sun.

TIP

The next round should send the left leg back first (as in step 6) and then continue with the opposite leg to the one used in the previous round.

TIPS

Gradually build up the number of rounds you can do. Begin with two rounds, then four, then six and so on.

Try to co-ordinate your breathing as you go. It will eventually come naturally as the postures themselves create a specific ebbing and flowing of the breath.

Traditionally, this sequence is practised at dawn, facing the sun as it rises.

To vary your daily routine you can alter:

– the breathing practice or pranayama technique (Simple Breathing, Sun Breath, Alternate Nostril Breathing or Bee Breath)

– posture sequence (Salute to the Sun or the sequence included in the 'Asanas' chapter)

– relaxation technique (Savasana, Relaxation 1 or 2, or Little Yoga Nidra).

As you become more used to a daily yoga routine, you can spend as little as 15 minutes to keep your body and mind healthy. You will, however, benefit a great deal more if you can set aside about an hour a day.

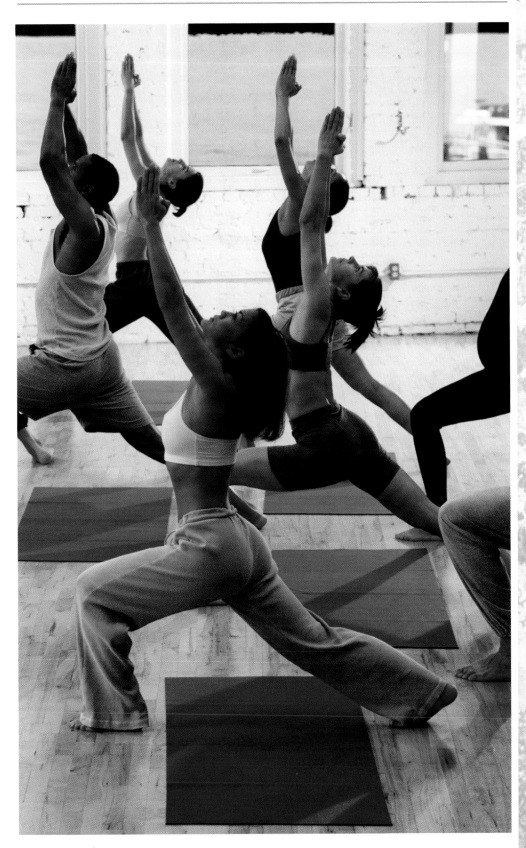

Left: Yoga being practised in a group.

MEDITATION

The traditional steps of pratyahara (sense withdrawal), dharana (concentration) and dhyana (meditation) tend to merge into one another. Meditation is, perhaps, one of the most misunderstood practices associated with spiritual development or religious devotion.

All of us fall into meditative states when our thought processes switch off from our normal conscious behaviour. Sitting beside a river, watching a sunset, or being immersed in a task we enjoy are all occasions when our focus shifts and we reach a point where our experience spontaneously changes.

Meditation is NOT a guided visualisation, a forced or strained process or an escape (by shutting off) from the world. It is a natural process that, when allowed to happen in a time and place set aside for the practice, gives our bodies the opportunity to heal and relax, for our mind to quieten and for our true self to perceive its place in the scheme of things.

Over thousands of years there have been many techniques developed that help us along with the process.

Right: a monk meditating.

Far right: meditation is a natural process that, when allowed to happen in a time and place set aside for the practice, gives our bodies the opportunity to heal and relax, for our mind to quieten and for our true self to perceive its place in the scheme of things.

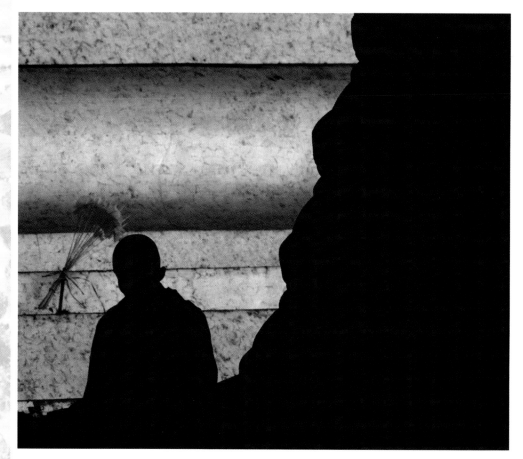

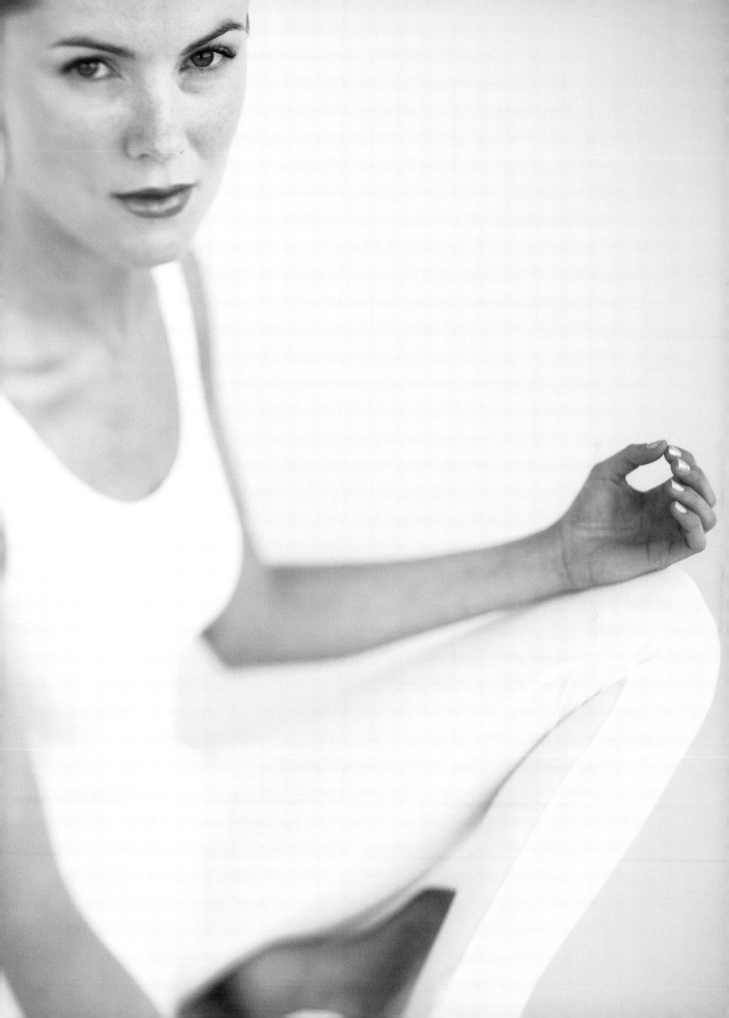

SETTING THE SCENE

Classically, meditation is practised at dawn and sunset, though any time of day is fine as long as it becomes a regular thing. It may take some while and several false starts before you can establish a practical routine for your lifestyle.

If one technique does not seem to "work", then try one of the others. Different people find different techniques work for them. There are no hard and fast rules. However, give yourself a good chance to settle down with each technique – don't expect everything to be easy right from the start.

1. Find a place where you can be comfortable, a clean, quiet spot, with maybe some flowers and items appropriate to your spiritual or religious inclinations.

2. Take steps to ensure you will have 5–20 minutes without interruption.

3. If you are sitting in a chair, place something under your feet if they do not easily reach the floor.

4. If you are sitting on the floor, ensure you have a blanket or mat, and maybe a cushion to place under the base of your spine. Your hips need to be higher than your knees and ankles for a posture that will not strain your hip joints.

5. If the weather is cool, then have a blanket or shawl close by to drape over your shoulders.

Right: Classical meditation is practised at dawn and sunset.

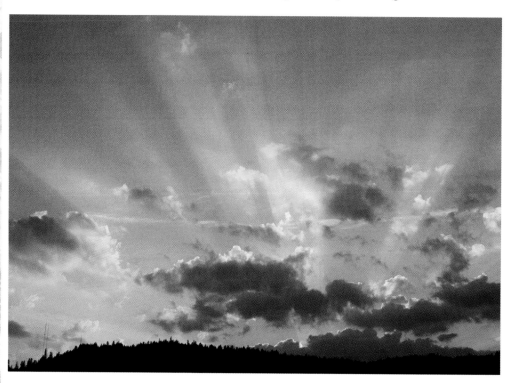

A few techniques for you to try:

USING THE BREATH

1 *Begin by preparing your meditation space so that you will be comfortable – setting the scene.*

2 *Practise a few rounds of a pranayama.*

3 *Switch your attention to your breathing in a more relaxed way.*

4 *Watch the breathing in and breathing out, without trying to control the breath in any way.*

5 *When you notice your attention has wandered, gently bring it back to the breath.*

6 *Continue until you are ready to come out of the meditation.*

TIPS

If you are meditating sitting on a cushion, you may want to make yourself a "gomtag" or meditation strap to help to support your back.

WHAT YOU NEED:
Strips of strong, inflexible fabric, (like canvas), the width of your fist with thumb extended and double the length of the distance from your finger tips, along the length of your arm, to the tip of your nose (head turned away from the arm you are measuring).

Sew the fabric into a large loop and tidy up the edges.

If you want a particular colour or design, you can cover the canvas with another more decorative fabric.

TO USE:
1. Rest the strap behind the lower back/top of hip bones and loop the rest over your knees.

2. Sit with your ankles crossed or with the soles of your feet together, knees apart. Adjust until you are comfortable.

"TRATAK"
Steady Gazing

Tratak or steady gazing is an excellent concentration and meditation exercise. Begin the process by gazing at an object, without blinking and then closing your eyes and visualising the object. It helps to steady the mind because the mind mirrors whatever the eyes do. Focusing on a single item or point helps the mind to do likewise.

Below: when practising steady gazing make sure the object is placed at eye level.

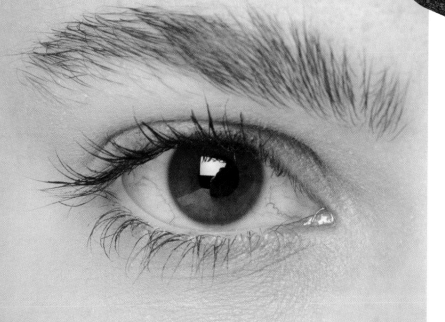

It is usually practised using a candle as a focus for the gaze, but you can use anything as a focus, like a flower or a stone. Begin by setting the scene and placing the item that you are going to gaze at.

1 Place the object at eye level about an arm's length away from you.

2 Settle your breathing, using a pranayama.

3 Open your eyes and look steadily at the item. Try not to strain.

4 After about a minute, close your eyes.

5 Visualise the item in your heart chakra (centre of the chest) or in your ajna chakra (centre of the forehead).

6 When the image fades, open your eyes and repeat.

Although this may at first cause your eyes to run, it actually improves your eyesight.

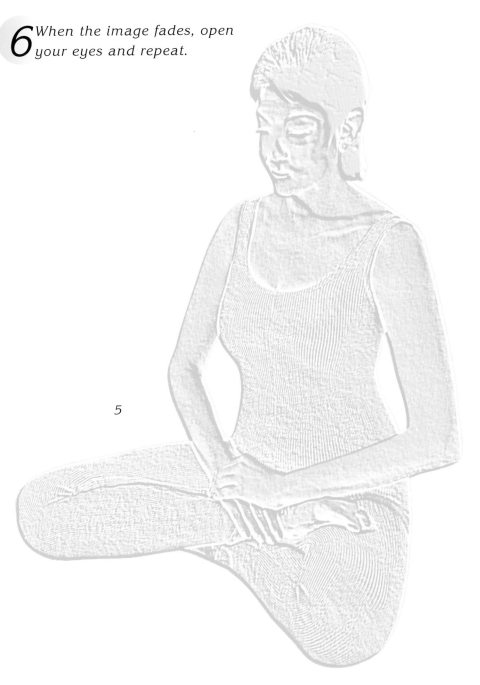

5

SOUND

Sound is used the world over as a means to alter states of awareness. Its effect can vary depending on the quality of the note. When linked with sacred words it can be a most effective meditation tool, known as mantra.

Prayers, hymns and chants are all examples of sound used for specific spiritual purposes. The ancient languages such as Latin and Sanskrit exert a lot of power in the actual sounds created by their words.

Many powerful words are related to well known belief systems. "Hail Mary", The Lord's Prayer and Psalm 23 are excellent examples within the Christian tradition; "Ram" and "Om Namah Shivaya" are from Hindu; and "Om Mani Padme Hum" and "A" are from Tibetan tradition.

The universal sound of AUM appears in various forms, apart from the original Sanskrit. It is "Amen" in Christianity and Judaism and "Amin" in Islam.

You can use sound out loud. It can be wonderfully effective in a group situation or when you have no worries about being overheard.

You can use sound whispered, or silently in your head. The most useful is probably a combination of these last two – allowing your lips to move, but with little or no sound being produced.

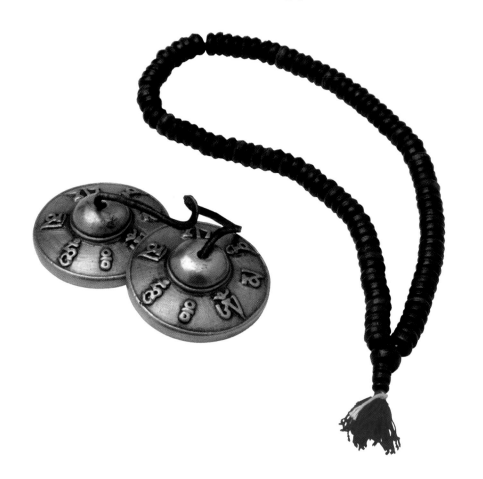

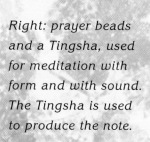

Right: prayer beads and a Tingsha, used for meditation with form and with sound. The Tingsha is used to produce the note.

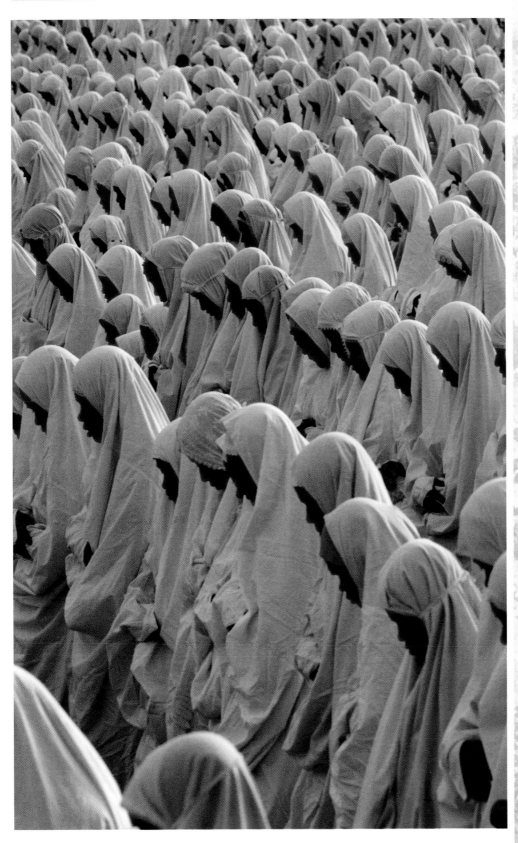

Left: Muslim women praying together.

Unless you have already chosen a sound to work with, try using AUM (pronounced Ooow-mmm) or A (pronounced Aaaaa).

1 *Begin by setting the scene.*

2 *Choose a sound you are comfortable with.*

3 *Begin with some pranayama.*

4 *Bring in the sound/mantra, initially sounding one on the out-breath, at a pitch and volume you are comfortable with.*

5 *Relax, and allow the sound/mantra and the breath to settle into a pattern that is right for you.*

6 *When you are ready to finish, just let the mantra fade away.*

Right: prayer beads, used during "meditation with form".

MALAS

Many traditions all over the world find value in keeping a count of how many mantras or prayers are said. Keeping count on the fingers can be done, but this brings the conscious mind into the meditation process. Keeping count by moving beads that are strung onto a thread is much easier and does not distract from the meditation process. These strings of beads are known by many names.

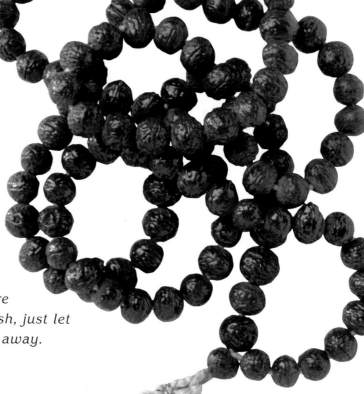

Malas, Tenghas, Rosaries or Prayer Beads

The most common number of beads on a thread is 108, but divisions of 108, like 54, or 27, are also found. In some traditions a few extra beads are added to represent specific mantras. When the beads are used in conjunction with a sound/mantra, one bead is moved along the string each time the word or phrase is spoken.

These three techniques are called "meditation with form".

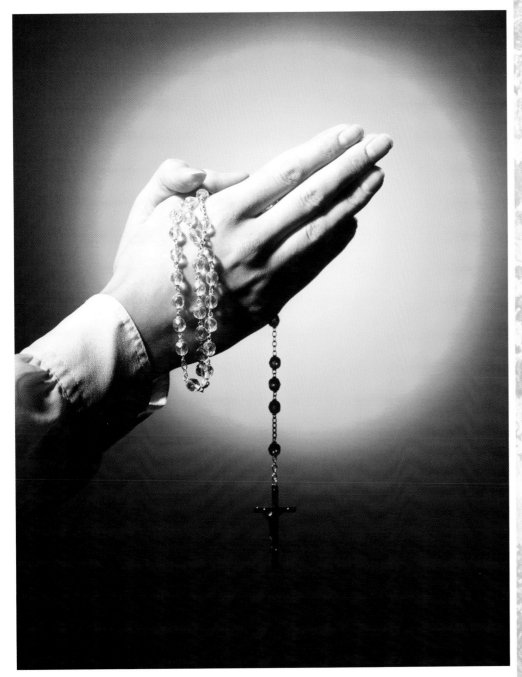

Left: a rosary being used during prayer.

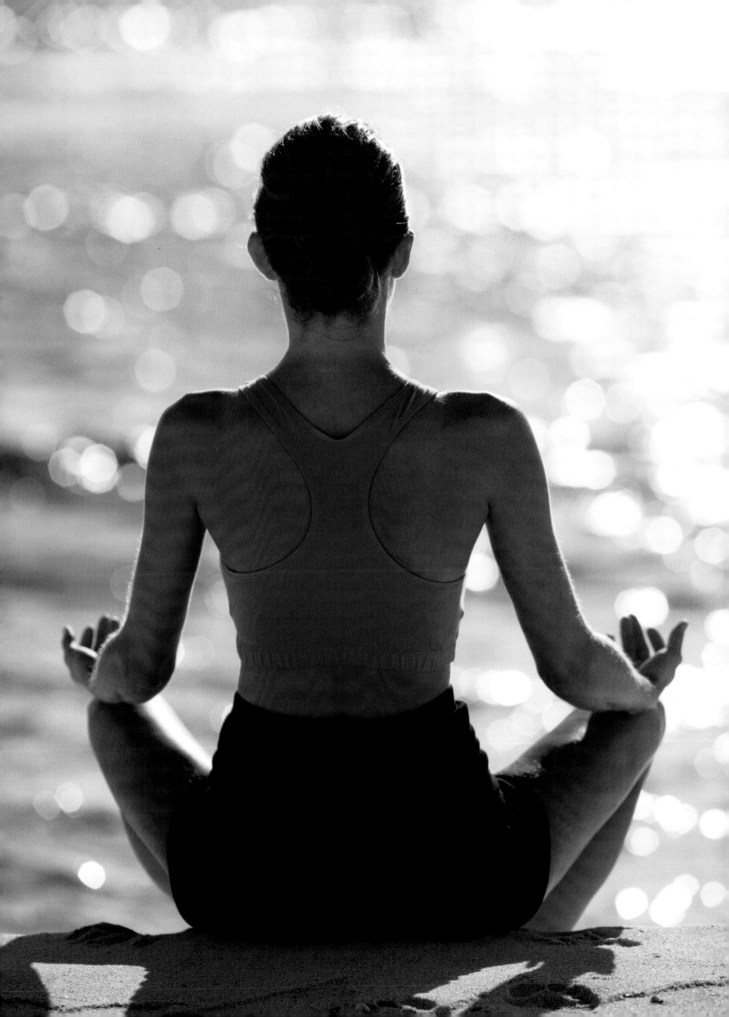

Meditation without form takes more time to develop, but can be explored by adapting the breathing meditation described earlier.

1 Begin by setting the scene.

2 Practice some pranayama, followed maybe by some mantra meditation.

3 Allow your mouth to open slightly, and also your eyes, so there is just a little light visible.

4 Switch your attention to your breathing, but only to the awareness of your breath as it passes in and out of your mouth. If there is focus anywhere, it is only on that.

5 Allow any thoughts that arrive to just go. Don't even acknowledge them.

6 If your mind wanders, gently bring your concentration back to the breath.

7 When you are ready to come out of meditation, open your eyes fully.

Note: if there is any sudden or loud noise, you will not jump because you are fully present and aware during the whole of the meditation process!

Far left: you can set the scene for meditation anywhere that you feel comfortable, and can find peace and quiet.

INDEX

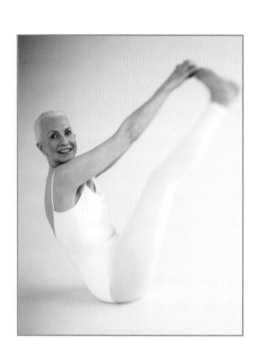